Virtual Clinical Excursions

for

Lewis, Heitkemper, and Dirksen:
MEDICAL-SURGICAL NURSING:
Assessment and Management of
Clinical Problems, 6th Edition

Virtual Clinical Excursions

for

Lewis, Heitkemper, and Dirksen:

MEDICAL-SURGICAL NURSING:
Assessment and Management of
Clinical Problems, 6th Edition

prepared by

Jean Foret Giddens, RN, PhD, CS

Virtual Clinical Excursions CD-ROM prepared by

Jay Shiro Tashiro, PhD, RN
Director of Systems Design
Wolfsong Informatics
Sedona, Arizona

Gina Long, RN, DNSc
Assistant Professor, Department of Nursing
College of Health Professions
Northern Arizona University
Flagstaff, Arizona

Ellen Sullins, PhD
Director of Research
Wolfsong Informatics
Sedona, Arizona

Michael Kelly, MS
Director of the Center for Research and
Evaluation of Advanced Technologies
in Education
Northern Arizona University
Flagstaff, Arizona

The development of Virtual Clinical Excursions Volume 1 was partially funded by the
National Science Foundation, under grant DUE 9950613.
Principal investigators were Tashiro, Sullins, Long, and Kelly.

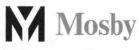

Mosby

An Affiliate of Elsevier Science
St. Louis   London   Philadelphia   Sydney   Toronto

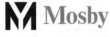
Mosby

An Affiliate of Elsevier Science

11830 Westline Industrial Drive
St. Louis, Missouri 63146

Virtual Clinical Excursions for   ISBN 0-323-02693-1
Lewis, Heitkemper, and Dirksen:
Medical-Surgical Nursing—Assessment and
Management of Clinical Problems,
6th Edition

NOTICE

Nursing is an ever-changing field. Standard safety precautions must be
followed, but as new research and clinical experience broaden our
knowledge, changes in treatment and drug therapy may become necessary or appropriate. Readers are advised to check the most current product information provided by the manufacturer of each drug to be administered to verify the recommended dose, the method and duration of
administration, and contraindications. It is the responsibility of the
licensed prescriber, relying on experience and knowledge of the patient,
to determine dosages and the best treatment for each individual patient.
Neither the publisher nor the author assumes any liability for any injury
and/or damage to persons or property arising from this publication.

The Publisher

Executive Vice President, Nursing & Health Professions: Sally Schrefer
Editor, Nursing: Tom Wilhelm
Senior Developmental Editor: Jeff Downing
Project Manager: Gayle May
Designer: Wordbench
Cover Art: Amy Buxton

WB

Printed in the United States of America

Last digit is the print number: 9 8 7 6 5 4 3 2 1

Workbook
prepared by

Jean Foret Giddens, RN, PhD, CS
Associate Professor, College of Nursing
University of New Mexico
Albuquerque, New Mexico

Textbook

Sharon Mantik Lewis, RN, PhD, FAAN
Professor, School of Nursing and Medicine
University of Texas Health Science Center
Clinical Nurse Scientist
Geriatric Research, Education, and Clinical Center
South Texas Veterans Health Care System
San Antonio, Texas

Margaret McLean Heitkemper, RN, PhD, FAAN
Professor, Biobehavioral Nursing and Health Systems
School of Nursing
Adjunct Professor, Division of Gastroenterology
School of Medicine
University of Washington
Seattle, Washington

Shannon Ruff Dirksen, RN, PhD
Associate Professor, College of Nursing
Arizona State University
Tempe, Arizona

Contents

Part VIII—Problems Related to Movement and Coordination

Getting Started

GETTING SET UP

■ MINIMUM SYSTEM REQUIREMENTS

Virtual Clinical Excursions is a hybrid CD, so it runs on both Macintosh and Windows platforms. To use *Virtual Clinical Excursions*, you will need one of the following systems:

- **Windows™**

    Windows 2000, 95, 98, NT 4.0
    IBM compatible computer
    Pentium II processor (or equivalent)
    300 MHz
    96 MB
    800 × 600 screen size
    Thousands of colors
    100 MB hard drive space
    12× CD-ROM drive
    Soundblaster 16 soundcard compatibility
    Stereo speakers or headphones

- **Macintosh®**

    MAC OS 9.04
    Apple Power PC G3
    300 MHz
    96 MB
    800 × 600 screen size
    Thousands of colors
    100 MB hard drive space
    12× CD-ROM drive
    Stereo speakers or headphones

Ideally, the system you use should have at least 200 MB of free disk space on your hard drive. There are commercially available desktop utility programs that can help clean up your hard drive. No other applications besides the operating system should be running at the time *Virtual Clinical Excursions* is running.

■ **INSTALLING** *VIRTUAL CLINICAL EXCURSIONS*

Virtual Clinical Excursions is designed to run from a set of files on your hard drive and a CD in your CD-ROM. Minimal installation is required.

● **Windows™**

1. Start Microsoft Windows and insert *Virtual Clinical Excursions* **Disk 1 (Installation)** in the CD-ROM drive.
2. Click the **Start** icon on the taskbar and select the **Run** option.
3. Type d:\setup.exe (where "d:\" is your CD-ROM drive) and press OK.
4. Follow the on-screen instructions for installation.
5. Remove *Virtual Clinical Excursions* **Disk 1 (Installation)** from your CD-ROM drive.
6. Restart your computer.

● **Macintosh®**

1. Insert *Virtual Clinical Excursions* **Disk 1 (Installation)** in the CD-ROM drive. The disk icon will appear on your desktop.
2. Double-click on the disk icon.
3. Double-click on the icon **Install Virtual Clinical Excursions**.
4. Follow the on-screen instructions for installation.
5. Remove *Virtual Clinical Excursions* **Disk 1 (Installation)** from your CD-ROM drive
6. Restart your computer.

■ **HOW TO ADJUST YOUR MONITOR'S SETTINGS (WINDOWS™ ONLY)**

● **Windows 95/98/SE/ME/2000**

1. Click the **Start** button and go to **Settings** on the pop-up menu. Click on **Control Panel**.
2. When the Control Panel window opens, double-click on the **Display** icon.
3. You will now be presented with the Display Properties window. Click on the **Settings** tab (on the right). Below the image of the monitor, you will see on the left the **Color** palette. (You should change this to **High Color [16 bit]** by selecting it from the drop-down menu. You will need to restart your computer to do this.) On the right is the desktop area. Left-click and hold down on the slider button and move it to 800 by 600 pixels. Now click **OK**.
4. Windows will ask you to confirm the change; click **OK**. Your screen will resize and Windows will again ask you whether you want to keep these new settings. Click **Yes**.

● **Windows XP**

1. Click the **Start** button; then click **Control Panel** on the pop-up menu.
2. Click **Display**. If Display does not appear, click **Switch to Classic View**; then click on **Display** icon.
3. From the Display Properties dialog box, select the **Settings** tab.
4. Under Screen Resolution, click and drag the sliding bar to adjust the desktop size to 800 x 600 pixels.
5. Under Color Quality, choose **High** or **Highest**.
6. Click **Apply**. If you approve of the new settings, click **Yes**.

■ HOW TO USE DISK 2 (PATIENTS' DISK)

- **Windows™**

  When you want to work with the five patients in the virtual hospital, follow these steps:

  1. Insert *Virtual Clinical Excursions* **Disk 2 (Patients' Disk)** into your CD-ROM drive.
  2. Double-click on the icon **Shortcut to Virtual Clinical Excursions**, which can be found on your desktop. This will load and run the program.

- **Macintosh®**

  When you want to work with the five patients in the virtual hospital, follow these steps:

  1. Insert *Virtual Clinical Excursions* **Disk 2 (Patients' Disk)** into your CD-ROM drive.
  2. Double-click on the icon **Shortcut to Virtual Clinical Excursions**, which can be found on your desktop. This will load and run the program.

■ QUALITY OF VISUALS, SPEED, AND COMMON PROBLEMS

Virtual Clinical Excursions uses the Apple QuickTime media layer system. This includes QuickTime Video and QuickTime VR Video, which allow for high-quality graphics and digital video. The graphics seen in the *Virtual Clinical Excursions* courseware should be of high quality with good color. If the movies and graphics appear blocky or otherwise low-quality, check to see whether your video card is set to "thousands of colors."

Note: Virtual Clinical Excursions is not designed to function at a 256-color depth. (You may need to go to the Control Panel and change the Display settings.) If you don't see any digital video options, please check that QuickTime is installed correctly.

The system should respond quickly and smoothly. In particular, you should not see any jerky motions or unannounced long delays as you move through the virtual hospital settings, interact with patients, or access information resources. If you notice slow, jerky, or delayed software responses, it may mean that your particular system requires additional RAM, your processor does not meet the basic requirements, or your hard drive is full or too fragmented. If the videos appear banded or subject to "breakup," you may need to find an updated video driver for the computer's video card. Please consult the manufacturer of the video card or computer for additional video drivers for your machine.

■ TECHNICAL SUPPORT

Technical support for this product is available at no charge by calling the Technical Support Hotline between 9 a.m. and 5 p.m. (Central Time), Monday through Friday. Inside the United States, call 1-800-692-9010. Outside the United States, call 314-872-8370.

A QUICK TOUR

Welcome to *Virtual Clinical Excursions*, a virtual hospital setting in which you can work with five complex patient simulations and also learn to access and evaluate the information resources that are essential for high-quality patient care.

The virtual hospital, Red Rock Canyon Medical Center, is a teaching hospital for Canyonlands State University. Within the medical center, you will work on a medical-surgical floor with a realistic architecture as well as access information resources. The floor plan in which the patient scenarios unfold is constructed from a model of a real medical center. The medical-surgical unit has:

- Five patient rooms (Room 302, Room 303, Room 304, Room 309, Room 310)
- A Nurses' Station (Room 312)
- A Supervisor's Office (Room 301)
- Two conference rooms (Room 307, Room 308)
- A nurses' lounge (Room 306)

■ BEFORE YOU START

Make sure you have your textbook nearby when you use the *Virtual Clinical Excursions Patients' Disk*. You will want to consult topic areas in your textbook frequently while working with the CD and using this workbook.

■ SUPERVISOR'S OFFICE (ROOM 301)

Just like a real-world clinical rotation, you have to let someone know when you arrive on the hospital floor—and you have to let someone know when you leave the floor. This process is completed in the Supervisor's Office (Room 301).

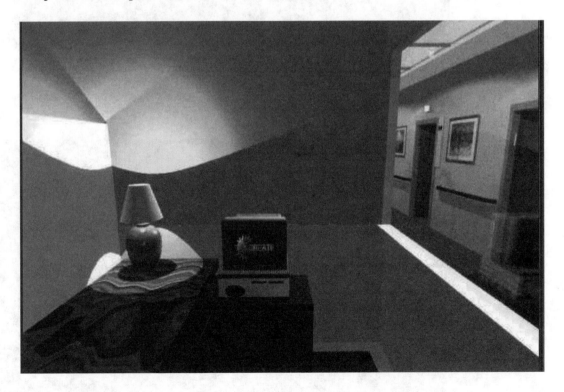

To get a 360° view of where you are "standing":

- Place the cursor in the middle of the screen.
- Hold down the mouse.
- Drag either right or left.

You will see you are in a room with an alcove to your left and a door behind you. To move into the hallway, place the cursor in the door opening and click. Once you are in the hallway, hold down the mouse and make a 360° turn.

In one direction, you will see:

- An exit sign
- An elevator
- A waiting room

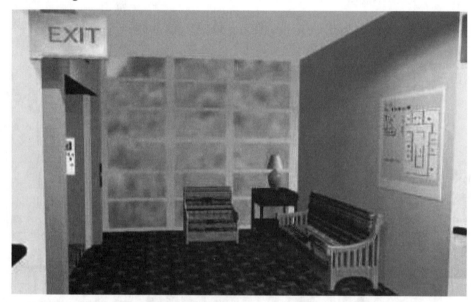

In the other direction, you will see a:

- Patient room
- Mobile computer

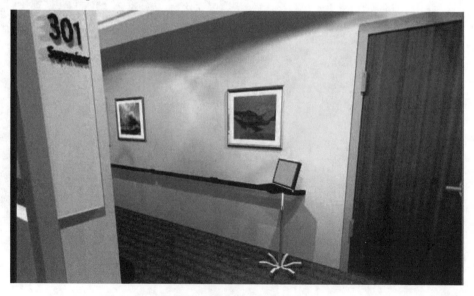

Move the cursor to a new place along the hallway outside the Supervisor's Office and click again. (Always try to place the cursor in the middle of the screen.) You should be moving along the hallway. Remember, at any point you can hold down the mouse and turn 360° in either direction. You can also hold down and move the mouse to the top or bottom of the frame, giving you views looking up or down.

■ READING ROOM

Go back into the Supervisor's Office by clicking on anything inside the room. Explore the Supervisor's Office (Room 301), and you will find another computer. This computer is a link to Canyonlands State University, the simulated university associated with the Red Rock Canyon Medical Center. Double-click on this computer, and a Web browser screen will be launched, which will open the Medical-Nursing Library in Canyonlands State University.

Click on the **Reading Room** icon, and you will see a table of icons that allows you to read short learning modules on a variety of anatomy and physiology topics.

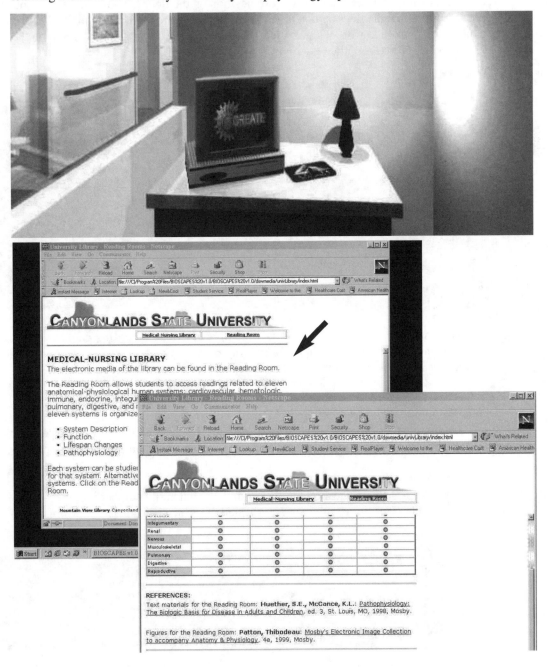

When you are ready to exit the reading room, go to the **File** icon on the browser, look at the drop-down menu, and select **Exit** or **Close**, depending on your Web browser. The browser will close, and once again you will be looking at the computer in the Supervisor's Office.

■ FLOOR MAP AND ANIMATED MAP

Move into the hallway outside the Supervisor's Office and turn right. A floor map can be found on the wall in the waiting area opposite the elevator and exit sign. To get there, click on anything in the waiting area. You should be able to see the map now, but you may not be close enough to open it. Click again on an object in the waiting area; this will move you closer. Turn to the right until you can see the map. Double-click on the map, and you will get a close-up view of the medical-surgical floor's layout. Click on the **Return** icon to exit this close-up view of the floor map.

Compare the floor map on the wall with the animated map in the upper right-hand corner of your screen. The green dot follows your position on the floor to show you where you are. You can move about the floor by double-clicking on the different rooms in this map. If you have already signed in to work with a patient, double-clicking on the patient's room on the animated map will take you right into the room.

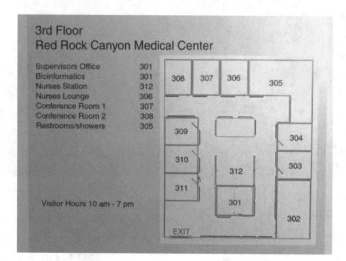
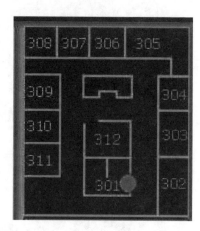

Note: If you have not signed in to work with a patient, double-clicking on a patient's room on the animated map will take you to the hallway right outside the room. If you have not yet selected a patient, you cannot access patient rooms or records.

■ HOW TO SIGN IN

To select a patient, you will need to sign in on the desktop computer in the Supervisor's Office (Room 301). Double-click on the computer screen, and a log-on screen will appear.

- Replace *Student Name* with your name.
- Replace the student ID number with your student ID number.
- Click **Continue** in the lower right side of the screen.

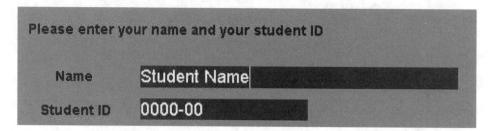

■ HOW TO SELECT A PATIENT

You can choose any one of five patients to work with. For each patient you can select either of two 4-hour shifts on Tuesday or Thursday (0700–1100 or 1100–1500). You can also select a Friday morning period in which you can review all of the data for the patient you selected. You will not, however, be able to visit patients on Friday, only review their records.

■ PATIENT LIST

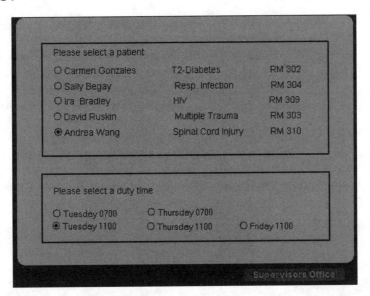

- **Carmen Gonzales (Room 302)**

  Diabetes mellitus, type 2 – An older Hispanic female with an infected leg that has become gangrenous. She has type 2 diabetes mellitus, as well as complications of congestive heart failure and osteomyelitis.

- **David Ruskin (Room 303)**

  Motor vehicle accident – A young adult African-American male admitted with a possible closed head injury and a severely fractured right humerus following a car-bicycle accident. He undergoes an open reduction and internal fixations of the right humerus.

- **Sally Begay (Room 304)**

  Respiratory infection – A Native American woman initially suspected to have a Hantavirus infection. She has a confirmed diagnosis of bacterial lung infection. This patient's complications include chronic obstructive pulmonary disease and inactive tuberculosis.

- **Ira Bradley (Room 309)**

  HIV-AIDS – A Caucasian adult male in late-stage HIV infection admitted for an opportunistic respiratory infection. He has complications of oral fungal infection, malnutrition, and wasting. Patient-family interactions also provide opportunities to explore complex psychosocial problems.

- **Andrea Wang (Room 310)**

  Spinal cord injury – A young Asian female who entered the hospital after a diving accident in which her T6 was crushed, with partial transection of the spinal cord. After a week in ICU, she has been transferred to the Medical-Surgical unit, where she is being closely monitored.

Note: You can select only one patient for one time period. If you are assigned to work with multiple patients, return to the Supervisor's Office to switch from one patient to another.

■ HOW TO FIND A PATIENT'S RECORDS

Nurses' Station (Room 312)

Within the Nurses' Station, you will see:

1. A blue notebook on the counter—this is the Medication Administration Record (MAR).
2. A bookshelf with patient charts.
3. Two desktop computers—the computer to the left of the bulletin board is used to access Red Rock Canyon Medical Center's Intranet; the computer to the right beneath the bookshelf is used to access the Electronic Patient Record (EPR). *(Note: You can also access the EPR from the mobile computer outside the Supervisor's Office, next to Room 302.)*
4. A bulletin board—this contains important information for students.

As you use these resources, you will always be able to return to the Nurses' Station (Room 312) by clicking either a **Nurses' Station** icon or a **3rd Floor** icon located next to the red cross in the lower right-hand corner of the computer screen.

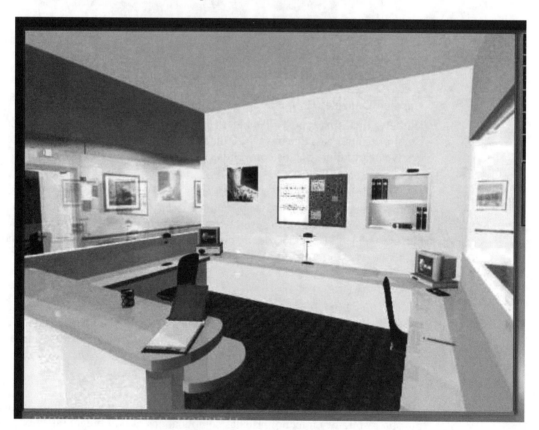

1. Medication Administration Record (MAR)

The blue notebook on the counter in the Nurses' Station (Room 312) is the Medication Adminis-tration Record (MAR), listing current 24-hour medications for each patient. Simply click on the MAR, and it opens like a notebook. Tabs allow you to select patients by room number. Each MAR sheet lists the following:

- Medications
- Route and dosage of medications
- Times of administration of medication

The MAR changes each day.

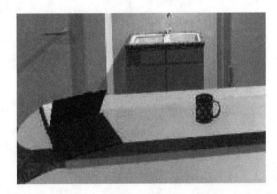

START	END	MEDICATION	2301 0700	0701 1500	1501 2300
		Cefoxitin, 2 g IVPB q6h	0300 *LG*	0900 *JS* 1500	2100
		Glyburide, 3.0 mg PO qA.M., with breakfast		0800 *JS*	
		Blood Glucose, AC and HS *0730 = 260, 1100 = 170*		0730 *JS* 1100 *JS*	
		Decrease D$_5$ 0.45 NS, 20 cc/hour	0600 *LG*		
		Morphine Sulfate, IM 2-5 mg q1-2h, PRN for severe pain *5mg @ 0300, 0600 LG* *5mg @ 0800*	0300 *LG* 0600 *LG*	0800 *JS*	

PATIENT: Gonzales, Carmen   MR# 20194873   DAY: Tuesday

118%   1 of 1   8 x 14 in

302   303   304   309   310

2. Charts

In the back right-hand corner of the Nurses' Station (Room 312) is a bookshelf with patient charts. To open a chart:

- Double-click on the bookshelf.
- Click once on the chart of your choice.

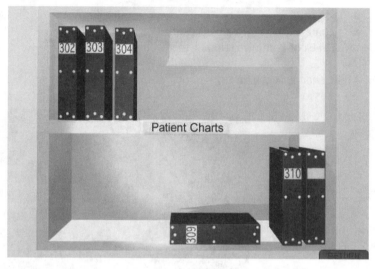

Tabs at the bottom of each patient's chart allow you to review the following data:

- Physical & History*
- Physicians' Notes
- Physicians' Orders
- Nurses' Notes
- Diagnostics Reports

- Expired MARs
- Health Team Reports
- Surgeons' Notes
- Other Reports

"Flip" forward by selecting a tab or backward by clicking on the small chart icon in the lower right side of your screen. (**Flip Back** appears on this icon once you have moved beyond the first tab.) As in the real world, the data in each patient's chart changes daily.

Note: Physical & History is a seven-page PDF file for Carmen Gonzales, David Ruskin, and Ira Bradley. Physical & History is a five-page PDF file for Andrea Wang and Sally Begay. Remember to scroll down to read all pages.

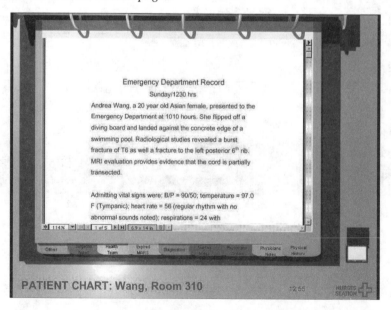

3. Two Computers

◆ **Electronic Patient Record (EPR)**

You can only access an Electronic Patient Record (EPR) once you have signed in and selected the patient in the Supervisor's Office (Room 301). The EPR can be accessed from two computers:

- Desktop computer under the bookshelf in the Nurses' Station (Room 312)
- Mobile computer outside the Supervisor's Office, next to Room 302

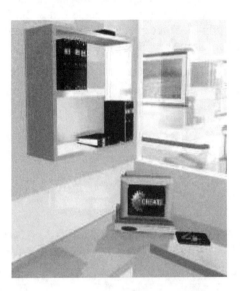 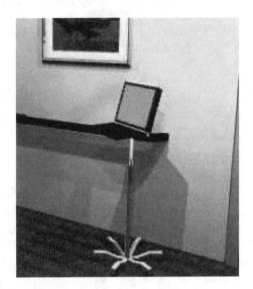

To access a patient's EPR:

- Double-click on the computer screen.
- Type in the password—it will always be **rn2b**.
- Click on **Access Records**.
- Click on the patient's name, then on **Access EPR** (or simply double-click on the patient's name).

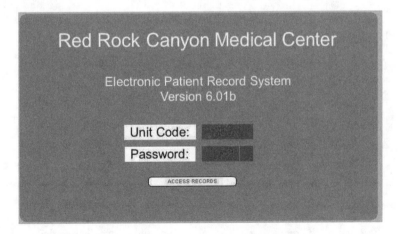

*Note: Do **not** press the Return/Enter key. If you make a mistake, simply delete the password, reenter it, and click Access Records. You will then enter the records system, where you find a list of patients.*

The EPR form represents a composite of commercial versions being used in hospitals and clinics. You can access the EPR:

- For a patient
- To review existing data
- To enter data you collect while working with a patient

The EPR is updated daily, so no matter what day or part of a shift you are working, there will be a current EPR with the patient's data from the past days of the current hospital stay. This type of simulated EPR allows you to examine how data for different attributes have changed over time, as well as to examine data for all of a patient's attributes at a particular time. The EPR is fully functional (as it is in a real-life hospital or clinic). You can enter such data as blood pressure, heart rate, and temperature. The EPR will not, however, allow you to enter data for a previous time period.

At the lower left corner of the EPR, there are nine icons that allow you to view different types of patient data:

- Assessment
- Admissions
- Urinanalysis
- Vital Signs
- ADL

- Blood Gases
- I&O
- Chemistry
- Hematology

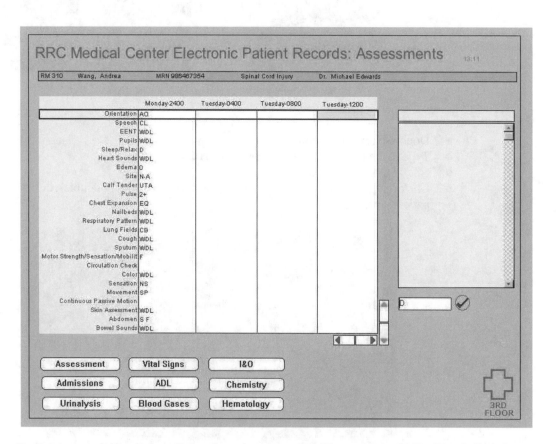

Remember, each hospital or clinic selects its own codes. The codes in the Red Rock Canyon Medical Center may be different from ones you have seen in clinical rotations that have computerized patient records.

You use the codes for the data type, selecting the code to describe your assessment findings and typing that code in the box in the lower right side of the screen, to the left of the checkmark symbol (✓).

Once the data are typed in this box, they are entered into the patient's record by clicking on the checkmark (✓). Make sure you are in the correct cell by looking for the placement of the blue box in the table. That box identifies which cell the database is "looking" at for any given moment.

You can leave the EPR by clicking on the **3rd Floor** icon in the lower right corner. This takes you back into the Nurses' Station (Room 312).

◆ Intranet

The computer on the left of the bulletin board in the Nurses' Station (Room 312) is dedicated to Red Rock Canyon Medical Center's **Intranet**. This system contains resources related to working within the hospital. Again, a double click on the screen will activate the computer. A Web browser will come up with four options (Hospital News, Employment, InfoStat, and Home). Navigate within the Intranet just as you would within a Web-based Internet site. Click on **Hospital News** and read some of the articles. The Employment icon opens a screen with descriptions of jobs available in the hospital. The InfoStat icon will connect the hospital Intranet to the Internet. *(Note: This option searches for your Internet connection, activates that connection, and takes you to the publisher's Website for your textbook.)* When in doubt, click on **Home**, which will take you back to the home page for the site.

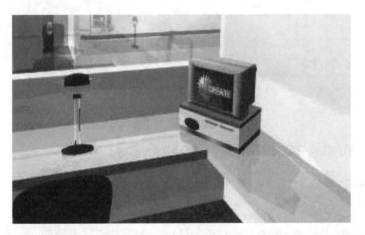

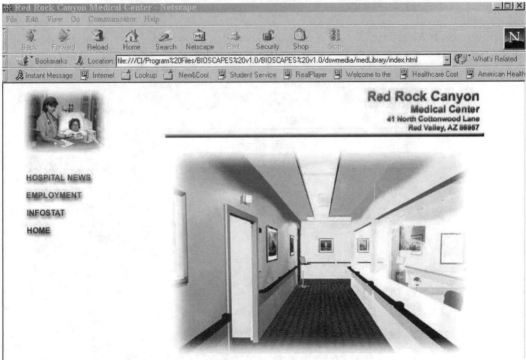

To return to the **Nurses' Station (Room 312)**, exit from the browser. This computer simulates being in a Web environment, so you have to exit from the Intranet by exiting from the browser. Click on **File**, then on **Exit** or **Close** (depending on your browser).

4. Bulletin Board

The bulletin board in the Nurses' Station (Room 312) has important information for students. Click on the board and you can read where reports are being given for patients and where the health team meetings are being held. Lessons in your workbook will direct you to these meetings and reports. Click on **Return** to exit this close-up view of the board.

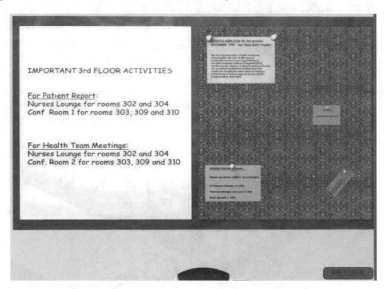

■ VISITING A PATIENT

First, go the Supervisor's Office and sign in to work with Andrea Wang for Tuesday at 0700. Now go to her room. *(Note: The quickest way to get to a patient's room is by double-clicking the room number on the animated map. You can also choose to move through the hallway until you reach the patient's door; then click on the doorknob.)* Once you are inside the room, you will see a still frame of your patient. Below this frame, you will find four icons:

- Vital Signs
- Health History
- Physical
- Medications

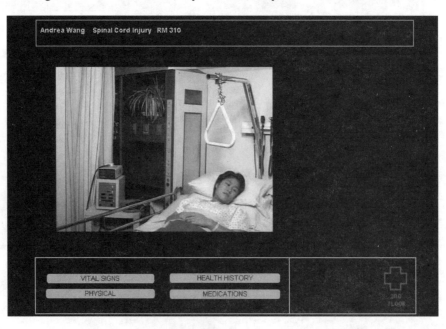

Each of these icons provides the opportunity to assess the patient or the patient's medications. When you click on an icon, you will follow a nurse through the process of collecting assessment data. The nurse will not speak to you but will rely on you to collect the data obtained during patient assessment, to record patient data in the EPR, and sometimes to make decisions after a nurse-patient interaction.

◆   **Vital Signs**

Click on **Vital Signs**; six new icons appear. Each of these new icons allows you to collect data for a particular vital sign. *(Note: You can also see two icons in the right corner.* **Continue Working with Patient** *takes you back to the main menu for this patient. Clicking on* **3rd Floor** *will take you back into the hallway.)* Click on the **Temperature** icon. You will see the nurse take the patient's temperature with a tympanic thermometer. At the end of the measurement, the temperature is shown in the animation of the thermometer to the right of the video screen. These types of interactions allow you to collect data during patient visits.

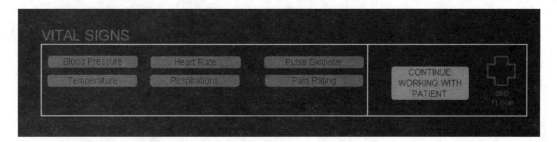

◆   **Physical Examination**

Click **Continue Working with Patient** to return to the main patient menu. Now click the **Physical** icon. Note the different areas of physical examination you can conduct. Try one.

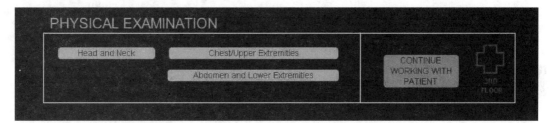

◆   **Health History**

Next, click **Continue Working with Patient** and select the **Health History** icon. In this interactive learning arena, you can ask the patient about her health history. Questions are organized into 12 categories, each of which is accessed by an icon below the video screen. Click on **Culture**, and three new icons appear in the frame to the right of the video. Click on the **Preferred Language** icon, and you will discover the language this patient prefers to use. For each of the 12 question areas, there are three topics you can explore. Thus, there are 36 different question areas related to the health history of each patient.

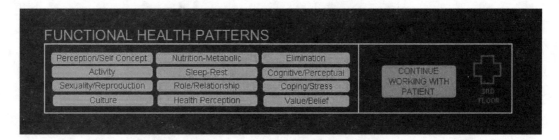

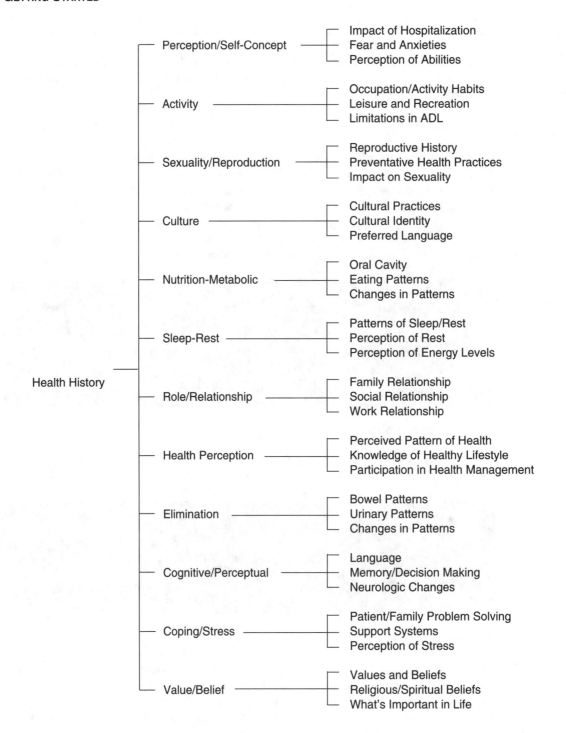

Health History

- Perception/Self-Concept
  - Impact of Hospitalization
  - Fear and Anxieties
  - Perception of Abilities
- Activity
  - Occupation/Activity Habits
  - Leisure and Recreation
  - Limitations in ADL
- Sexuality/Reproduction
  - Reproductive History
  - Preventative Health Practices
  - Impact on Sexuality
- Culture
  - Cultural Practices
  - Cultural Identity
  - Preferred Language
- Nutrition-Metabolic
  - Oral Cavity
  - Eating Patterns
  - Changes in Patterns
- Sleep-Rest
  - Patterns of Sleep/Rest
  - Perception of Rest
  - Perception of Energy Levels
- Role/Relationship
  - Family Relationship
  - Social Relationship
  - Work Relationship
- Health Perception
  - Perceived Pattern of Health
  - Knowledge of Healthy Lifestyle
  - Participation in Health Management
- Elimination
  - Bowel Patterns
  - Urinary Patterns
  - Changes in Patterns
- Cognitive/Perceptual
  - Language
  - Memory/Decision Making
  - Neurologic Changes
- Coping/Stress
  - Patient/Family Problem Solving
  - Support Systems
  - Perception of Stress
- Value/Belief
  - Values and Beliefs
  - Religious/Spiritual Beliefs
  - What's Important in Life

◆   **Medications**

Click **Continue Working with Patient**, and then click the **Medications** icon. Notice that you have three options within this learning environment: Review Medications, Administer, and Hold Medications. Don't click on these now, because you will need to look at this patient's records before you decide whether or not to give medications.

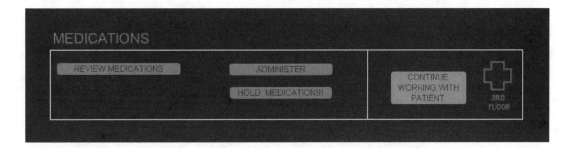

■ HOW TO QUIT OR CHANGE PATIENTS

How to Quit: If necessary, click either the **3rd Floor** icon or the **Nurses' Station** icon (depending on which screen you are currently using) to return to the medical-surgical floor. Then click on the **Quit** icon in the lower right corner of your screen.

How to Change Patients or Shifts: Go to the Supervisor's Office and double-click on the sign-in computer. Click the **Reset** icon. When the next screen appears, select a new patient or a different shift with the same patient.

A DETAILED TOUR

If you wish to understand the capabilities of the virtual hospital, take a detailed tour by going through the following section.

■ WORKING WITH A PATIENT

Sign in and select Carmen Gonzales as your patient for Tuesday at 0700 hours.

To become more familiar with the *Virtual Clinical Excursions Patients' Disk,* try the following exercises. These activities are designed to introduce you to all of the different components and learning opportunities available within the software. Each exercise will ask you to collect data on a patient.

■ REPORT

In hospitals, when one nurse's shift ends and another begins, the outgoing nurse who attended a patient will give a verbal and sometimes a written summary of that patient's condition to the incoming nurse who will assume care for the patient. This summary is called a *report* and is an important source of data to provide an overview of a patient.

Your first task is to get the report on Carmen Gonzales. Go to the bulletin board in the Nurses' Station. Double-click on the board and check the location where the attending nurse from the previous shift will give you report on this patient. Remember, Carmen Gonzales is in Room 302, so look for that room number on the bulletin board. You will find that the report is being given in the Nurses' Lounge (Room 306). Click **Return** to leave this close-up view of the bulletin board. *(Note: You can also find out where reports are being given by moving your cursor across the animated map.)* Go to Room 306 by double-clicking on the animated map. Once inside the room, click on **Report** and then on **Gonzales**. Listen to report and make a list of this patient's problems and high-priority concerns. When you are finished, click on the **3rd Floor** icon to return to the Nurses' Station.

Problems/Concerns

■ CHARTS

Find the patient charts in the bookshelf to the right of the bulletin board. Double-click on the bookshelf and find Carmen Gonzales' chart (the one labeled **302**). Click on her chart and read the section called Physical & History, including the Emergency Department Record. Determine from this information why Carmen Gonzales has been admitted to the hospital. In the space below, write a brief summary of why this patient was admitted.

■ MEDICATIONS

Open the Medication Administration Record (MAR) by clicking on the blue notebook on the counter of the Nurses' Station. Find the list of medications prescribed for Carmen Gonzales, and write down the medications that need to be given during the time period 0730–0930. For each medication, note dosage, route, and time in the chart below.

Time	Medication	Dosage	Route

Close the MAR and go inside Carmen Gonzales' room (302). Click on the **Medications** icon. You will be responsible for administering the medications ordered during the time period 0730–0930.

To become familiar with the medication options, look at the frame below the video screen. There you will find three opportunities:

- Review Medications
- Administer
- Hold Medications

Click on **Review Medications**. This brings up a frame to the right of the video screen with a list of the medications ordered for the period 0730–0930 hours. Decide whether these medications match what appears within the **Medication Administration Record (MAR)** for this time period. If they do match, you can click the **Administer** icon. If they do not match, you should select **Hold Medications**. When you are finished, click **Continue Working With Patient** to return to the patient care menu.

■ VITAL SIGNS

Vital signs are often considered the traditional signs of life and include body temperature, heart rate, respiratory rate, blood pressure, oxygen saturation of the blood, and the patient's experience of pain.

Inside Carmen Gonzales' room, click on the **Vital Signs** icon. This icon activates a pathway that allows you to measure the patient's vital signs. When you enter this pathway, you will see a short video in which the nurse informs the patient what is about to happen. Six vital signs options appear at the bottom of the screen. Each icon activates a video clip in which the respective vital sign is measured. Relevant vital signs data become available in these videos. For example, click on **Heart Rate**, and a video clip and animation of a radial pulse appear. You can measure the heart rate by counting the animated pulses during a prescribed time.

Try each of the different vital signs options to see what kinds of data are obtained. The vital signs data change over time to reflect the temporal changes you would find in a patient similar to Carmen Gonzales. You will see this most clearly if you "leave" the Tuesday time period you are currently within and "come back" on Thursday. However, you will also find changes throughout any given day (for example, differences between the 0700–1100 and 1100–1500 shifts).

Collect vital signs data for Carmen Gonzales and enter them into the following table. Note the time at which you collected these data.

Vital Signs	Findings/Time
Blood Pressure	
O$_2$ Saturation	
Heart Rate	
Respiratory Rate	
Temperature	
Pain Rating	

After you are done, click on the **3rd Floor** icon in the lower right portion of your screen. This will take you back into the hallway. Move along the hallway (or use the animated map in the upper right corner of your screen) to return to the Nurses' Station. Enter the station, and click on the computer that accesses the Electronic Patient Record (EPR). First you will see the Electronic Patient Record System entry screen. Type in **rn2b** for the password (remember, do *not* press the Return/Enter key). Then click **Access Records**, and you will see a new screen with patients listed. Click on **Carmen Gonzales** and then on **Access EPR**. Now you are in the EPR system. Click on **Vital Signs**, which will open the screen with vital signs data. Use the blue and orange arrows in the lower right-hand corner of the data table to move around within the database. Look at the data collected earlier for each of the vital signs you measured. Use these data to establish a baseline for each of the vital signs.

a. Are any of the data you collected signifi-cantly different from the baselines for those vital signs?	Circle One: Yes No
b. If "Yes," which data are different?	

■ PHYSICAL ASSESSMENT

After examining the EPR for vital signs, click the **Assessment** icon and review Carmen Gonzales' data in this area. Once you have reviewed the data and noted any areas of concern to you, close the EPR, enter Carmen Gonzales' room, and click on the **Physical** icon. This will activate the following three options for conducting a physical assessment of the patient:

- Head and Neck
- Chest/Upper Extremities
- Abdomen and Lower Extremities

Click on the **Head and Neck** icon. You will see the nurse conduct an assessment of the head and neck. At the end of the video, a series of icons appear in a frame to the right of the video screen. These icons list the different areas of the head and neck that were examined and the data obtained during the examination. The icons allow you to replay that section of the video in which the particular area was examined.

For example, if you click on **Oculomotor** (the finding is "Oculomotor function intact"), you will see a replay of the assessment of oculomotor function. Each of the icons activates only that portion of the head and neck assessment focused on the particular area described by the icon. The intention is to help you correlate each part of a physical assessment with the data obtained from that assessment—and to give you the opportunity to have the whole assessment of a region conducted beginning to end so that you can learn the process as well as its component parts. Click **Continue Working with Patient** and explore the Chest/Upper Extremities and the Abdomen and Lower Extremities options. For each area, browse through the icons that provide data on a particular area of the assessment. *(Note: The data for certain attributes found during physical assessments change for some patients as you follow them through the virtual week.)*

Focus on the examination of the abdomen and lower extremities by clicking on the option. Pay close attention to the leg wound. In the following table, record the data collected by the nurse during the examination.

Area of Examination	Findings
Abdomen	
Legs	

After you have completed the physical examination of the abdomen and lower extremities, click **Continue Working with Patient** to return to the patient care menu. From there, click on the **3rd Floor** icon and return to the Nurses' Station. Enter the data you collected in Carmen Gonzales' EPR. Compare the data that were already in the record with the data you just collected.

a. Are any of the data you collected significantly different from the baselines for those vital signs?	Circle One: Yes No
b. If "Yes," which data are different?	

■ HEALTH HISTORY

Conduct part of a health history of Carmen Gonzales. Return to her room and click on the **Health History** icon. Twelve health history areas become visible as icons below the video screen. For example, you can see Perception/Self-Concept, Activity, Sexuality/Reproduction, and so on. Note that this patient speaks Spanish and that the nurse has brought in a translator. All of the health history conversations with Carmen Gonzales are completed through translation. Clicking on any of the 12 health history icons reveals three question areas for that category. For example, if you click **Perception/Self-Concept**, a box appears to the right of the video screen with three question areas:

- Impact of Hospitalization
- Fear and Anxieties
- Perception of Abilities

Each of these three areas can be activated by clicking on their respective icons. When an icon is clicked, you will see a video in which your preceptor asks a question in the respective area and the patient answers through the translator.

Since there are 12 health history areas, with three areas of questioning for each, you have access to a total of 36 video clips that provide an opportunity to learn quite a bit about Carmen Gonzales. The questions and responses were chosen for reasons. In fact, conducting an actual health history would not unfold in such discrete and isolated moments; in the real world you would need to follow up some responses with additional questions. Other lessons in this workbook will encourage you to look at each of the health history areas and decide what additional questions need to be asked.

Unlike the vital signs and physical examination findings, the health history data do not change. The developers of *Virtual Clinical Excursions* realized that the number of videos (and the space required for storage) would become too large for the type of educational package we envisioned. We therefore decided to produce only one set of health history data-collecting opportunities. In truth, the health history would probably not change much over a week. Lessons in your workbook may have you collect health history data on the first day of care, or some of the health history queries may be assigned for Tuesday and the others for Thursday.

We recommend that you explore the health history of Carmen Gonzales by choosing some of the 12 categories and asking one or two of the three questions available for each area. When you are done exploring the health history options, leave the patient's room and go to one of the computers that allow you to access the EPR. Browse through the different data fields to see where you would enter data from the health history questions.

Remember: When you are ready to stop working with your *Virtual Clinical Excursions Patients' Disk*, click on the **Quit** icon found in the lower right-hand corner of any of the 3rd floor screens.

■ COLLECTING AND EVALUATING DATA

Each of the patient care activities generates a great deal of assessment data. Remember that after you collect data, you can go to the Nurses' Station or the mobile computer outside Room 302 and enter the data into the EPR. You also can review the data in the EPR, as well as review a patient's chart and MAR. You will get plenty of practice collecting and then evaluating data in the context of the patient's course during previous shifts.

Now, here's an important question for you:

> Did the previous sequence of exercises provide the most efficient way to assess Carmen Gonzales?

For example, you went to the patient's room to get vital signs, then back to the EPR to enter data and compare your finding with extant data. Then, you went back to the patient's room to do a physical examination, and again back to the EPR to enter and review data. If this back-and-forth process of data collection and recording seemed inefficient, remember the following:

- You want to plan all of your nursing activities to maximize efficiency while at the same time optimizing quality of patient care.
- You collect a tremendous amount of data when you work with a patient. Very few people can accurately remember all these data for more than a few minutes. Develop efficient assessment skills, and enter assessment data as soon as possible after collecting them.
- Assessment data are only the starting point for the nursing process.

Make a clear distinction between these first exercises and how you actually provide nursing care. These initial exercises were designed to involve you actively in the use of different software components. This workbook focuses on sensible practices for implementing the nursing process in ways that ensure the highest quality care of patients.

Most importantly, remember that a human being changes through time—and that these changes include both the physical and psychosocial facets of a person as a living organism. Think about this for a moment. Some patients may change physically in a very short time (a patient with emerging myocardial infarction) or more slowly (a patient with chronic illness). Patients' overall physical and psychosocial conditions may improve or deteriorate. They may have effective coping skills and familial support or feel they are alone and full of despair. In fact, each individual is a complex mix of physical and psychosocial elements, and at least some of these elements usually change through time.

Thus it is crucial *not* to think of the nursing process as a simple one-time, five-step procedure:

- Assessment
- Nursing Diagnosis
- Planning
- Implementation
- Evaluation

Rather, it is a creative and systematic approach to delivering nursing care. Furthermore, because all living organisms are constantly changing, we must apply the nursing process over and over. Each time we follow the nursing process for an individual patient, we refine our understanding of that patient's physical and psychosocial conditions based on collection and analyses of many different types of data. *Virtual Clinical Excursions* will help you develop both the creativity and the systematic approach needed to become a nurse who can deliver the highest quality care to all patients.

The following icons are used throughout the workbook to help you quickly identify particular activities and assignments:

 Indicates a reading assignment—tells you which textbook chapter(s) you should read before starting each lesson

 Indicates a writing activity

 Marks the beginning of an interactive CD-ROM activity—signals you to open or return to your *Virtual Clinical Excursions Patients' Disk*

 Indicates additional CD-ROM instructions

 Indicates questions and activities that require you to consult your textbook

The Continuum of Patient Care

∞ **Reading Assignment:** Community-Based Nursing and Home Care (Chapter 6)
Patients: Sally Begay, Room 304
Ira Bradley, Room 309
Andrea Wang, Room 310

In this lesson we will compare the hospital admissions and discharges of three different patients within the framework of the care continuum and from the standpoint of discharge needs. Before you begin, let's consider the term *acute care setting*. This term refers to care provided to acutely ill patients who are unable to care for themselves at home or within the community setting. These patients' needs require that they receive specialized medical and nursing care within a hospital setting. There are various types of units within an acute care hospital setting.

Critical Care—Critical care encompasses intensive care units and trauma and emergency care services. Patients most often cared for in these types of units have multiple complex physiologic needs, severe illness, or trauma. Care is highly focused, often involving life-supportive care and hemodynamic monitoring.

Observation Unit—An observation unit is also frquently referred to as a "step-down" unit. This type of unit encompasses care for patients who require frequent monitoring and more intensive care than that provided in a general nursing unit but who are not in need of critical care placement. A telemetry unit is a type of observation unit.

General Nursing Unit—Care in this type of setting is provided to patients who typically have acute episodes of a chronic medical condition or who require care for a new condition. These individuals are not in need of advanced monitoring or life-supportive care.

CD-ROM Activity

You will now conduct a brief medical record review of three patients: Sally Begay, Ira Bradley, and Andrea Wang. Open your *Virtual Clinical Excursions Patients' Disk*. First, go to the Supervisor's Office and sign in to work with Sally Begay on Thursday at 1100. Next, go to the Nurses' Station and find Sally Begay's chart. Click on the chart to open it.

- Read the entire Physical & History. (Remember to scroll down to read all pages.)
- Click on **Physicians' Orders**. Read the initial admission orders on Saturday at 1230. Note where the patient was admitted. When you are finished, click on the **Nurses' Station** icon to close the chart.

Student Notes

→ Go back to the Supervisor's Office. This time, sign in to work with Ira Bradley on Thursday at 1100. Next, go to the Nurses' Station and open his chart.

- Read the entire Physical & History, including the Emergency Department Report.
- Click on **Physicians' Orders**. Read the initial admission orders for Sunday at 2255. Note where the patient was admitted. When you are through, close the chart.

Student Notes

→ Return to the Supervisor's Office and sign in to work with Andrea Wang on Thursday at 1100. Next, go to the Nurses' Station and open Andrea Wang's chart.

- Read the entire Physical & History, including the Emergency Department Record.
- Click on **Health Team** and read the notes provided by the nurse case manager, Sara Terney. Note where the patient was originally admitted. When you are through, close the chart.

Student Notes

Answer the following questions based on what you found from your chart review.

1. Which patient was admitted to the critical care unit? (Circle one.)

    Sally Begay   Ira Bradley   Andrea Wang

2. Consider the description of acute care units on page 29. What data did you find in the admission orders and the Physical & History that justify this patient's admission to a critical care unit?

3. Which patient was admitted to the observation unit (telemetry)? (Circle one.)

    Sally Begay   Ira Bradley   Andrea Wang

4. Consider the description of observation units in the matching activity on page 29. What data exist in the admission orders and the Physical & History that justify this patient's admission to this type of unit?

5. Which patient was admitted to a general nursing unit? (Circle one.)

   Sally Begay   Ira Bradley   Andrea Wang

6. Consider the description of general nursing units in the matching activity on page 29. What data exist in the admission orders and the Physical & History that justify this patient's admission to this type of unit?

 Next, consider the content presented in your textbook regarding transitional care settings, long-term care settings, and home care settings. Specifically, review the terms *transitional care*, *long-term care*, and *home care*.

 7. Write a brief description of each of the following terms based on what you have read in your textbook.

Transitional care settings:

• Subacute care:

- Acute rehabilitation care:

- Long-term acute care:

Long-term care settings:

- Skilled nursing facilities:

- Intermediate care facilities:

Home health care settings:

- Hospice care:

→ Now consider the discharge needs of the three patients. First, go to the Supervisor's Office and sign in to work with Sally Begay on Thursday at 1100. Next, go to the Nurses' Station and open her chart.

- Click on **Health Team** and read the reports of the nurse case manager, the clinical nurse specialist, and the social worker. As you read, keep in mind possible discharge needs.

8. Based on what you have read in the health team report, which of the following—if ordered upon discharge from the acute care setting—would most likely benefit Sally Begay?

___ Subacute care

___ Acute rehabilitation care

___ Home care

___ Hospice care

9. In what way does Sally Begay fit the criteria for this need, based on what you identified from the description in the textbook?

→ Go back to the Supervisor's Office and sign in to work with Ira Bradley on Thursday at 1100. Next, go to the Nurses' Station and open his chart.

- Click on **Health Team** and read the reports of the nurse case manager, the clinical nurse specialist, and the social worker. As you read, keep in mind possible discharge needs.

10. Based on what you have read in the health team report, which of the following—if ordered upon discharge from the acute care setting—would most likely benefit Ira Bradley?

____ Subacute care

____ Acute rehabilitation care

____ Home care

____ Hospice care

11. In what way does Ira Bradley fit the criteria for this need, based on what you identified from the description in the textbook?

→ Go back to the Supervisor's Office and sign in to work with Andrea Wang on Thursday afternoon. Next, go to the Nurses' Station and open her chart.

- Click on **Health Team** and read the reports of the nurse case manager, the clinical nurse specialist, and the social worker. As you read, keep in mind possible discharge needs.

12. Based on what you have read in the health team report, which type of nursing care is being planned for Andrea Wang upon discharge from the acute care setting?

____ Subacute care

____ Acute rehabilitation care

____ Home care

____ Hospice care

13. In what way does Andrea Wang fit the criteria for this need, based on what you identified from the description in the textbook?

 14. Read the discussion of case management in the textbook. What does the term *case management* mean?

Overview

15. Consider any or all of the health team reports you read. How does the health team report of the nurse case manager differ from the clinical specialist's report and the social worker's report? Compare and contrast the differences among the three reports.

Focus of the Nurse Case Manager

Focus of the Clinical Nurse Specialist

Focus of the Social Worker

Culturally Competent Care

 Reading Assignment: Culturally Competent Care (Chapter 2)
Patients: Carmen Gonzales, Room 302
Sally Begay, Room 304

For this lesson, you will be working with two patients of different cultures. The goal of this lesson is to compare and contrast ethnic and cultural data for these individuals.

Writing Activity

Match each of the following terms with the corresponding description.

1. _____	Set of rules that serves as the basis for beliefs, attitudes, and behaviors by which individuals, groups, and communities live	a. Culture
		b. Ethnicity
2. _____	The integration of knowledge, attitudes, and skills that enable a nurse to provide culturally appropriate health care	c. Values
		d. Acculturation
3. _____	Refers to groups of individuals who share a common social and cultural heritage that is passed on through the generations and involves identification with the group	e. Assimilation
		f. Cultural competence
		g. Cultural awareness
4. _____	A process in which people lose their own cultural identity as they adopt and incorporate aspects of the prevailing culture	h. Cultural knowledge
5. _____	A process that involves understanding the key aspects of a cultural group, particularly in relation to health and health care practices	
6. _____	A term used to describe the knowledge, values, beliefs, art, morals, law, customs, and habits of members within a society	
7. _____	A process whereby members of one culture modify their own culture as a result of contact with another culture	
8. _____	A conscious learning process in which individuals become appreciative of and sensitive to the cultures of other people; an important step in providing culturally appropriate care and avoiding ethnocentrism	

Review Table 2-3 in your textbook. This table presents data you might include in a cultural assessment. Use this table as a guide to evaluate data collected for Carmen Gonzales and Sally Begay.

CD-ROM Activity

9. Go to the Supervisor's Office and sign in to work with Carmen Gonzales for the Tuesday 0700 shift. Go to Carmen Gonzales' room, click on **Health History**, and systematically go through all the available question areas. As you go through the history, identify parts of the history that form the cultural assessment. Fill in data as applicable in the table below.

When you have finished, return to the Supervisor's Office and sign in to work with Sally Begay for the Tuesday 0700 shift. Go to Sally Begay's room, click on **Health History**, and complete her portion of the table below.

Assessment	Carmen Gonzales	Sally Begay
Cultural group		
Values orientation		
Cultural sanctions and restrictions		
Communication		
Health-related beliefs and practices		
Nutrition		
Socioeconomic considerations		
Religious and spiritual considerations		

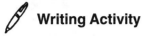 **Writing Activity**

10. Based on the data collected, what additional questions for Carmen Gonzales would help you further develop cultural awareness?

 Review Table 2-7 in the textbook and answer the following questions.

11. In what way was the use of an interpreter for Carmen Gonzales consistent with the suggestions in Table 2-7?

12. Did you identify anything that could have made the communication exchange better? If so, what?

Health History and Physical Examination— Part I

 Reading Assignment: Health History and Physical Examination (Chapter 3)
Patient: Sally Begay, Room 304

 This lesson will introduce you to the nursing history. Perhaps you have covered this content in another course. If so, this lesson will be valuable to you as a review. To begin, answer the following questions based on the reading from your textbook.

Writing Activity

1. What is the primary purpose of conducting a nursing history and physical examination?

2. How does a medical history differ from a nursing history?

3. What is the difference between subjective data and objective data?

4. What are the various sources of subjective data for a given patient?

The nursing history presented in the textbook is based on functional health patterns. Match each of the following descriptions or types of data with the corresponding functional health pattern. Refer to your textbook for help. (Answers may be used more than once.)

Description or Type of Data	Functional Health Pattern
5. _____ Identification of current stresses	a. Health Perception/ Health Management
6. _____ Focus on personal relationships	
7. _____ Body image and self-description	b. Nutrition/Metabolic
8. _____ Spiritual or religious preferences	c. Elimination
9. _____ Capacity to learn; how patient learns best	d. Activity/Exercise
10. _____ Practice of health habits and ways the patient stays healthy	e. Sleep/Rest
11. _____ Energy needed to carry out daily activities.	f. Cognitive/Perceptual
12. _____ Onset of menarche or menopause	g. Self-Perception/ Self-Concept
13. _____ Family history	h. Role/Relationship
14. _____ Condition of skin and ability for wounds to heal	i. Sexuality/Reproductive
15. _____ Questions related to the ability to see and hear	j. Coping/Stress Tolerance
16. _____ Identification of known risk factors for disease	k. Value/Belief
17. _____ Questions regarding recent losses or changes	
18. _____ Pattern of urinary and bowel elimination	
19. _____ Personal role or roles in life	
20. _____ Questions regarding ability to perform activities of daily living	
21. _____ Amount of sleep and degree of rest a patient experiences	
22. _____ Questions regarding oral intake and food preferences	
23. _____ Cultural preferences or values	
24. _____ Questions regarding pain	
25. _____ Methods of contraception and facilitation of conception	
26. _____ Questions regarding adherence to prescribed therapy	
27. _____ Questions about condition of teeth and ability to chew foods	
28. _____ Patient's feelings about the worth of life and health	

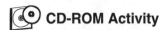 **CD-ROM Activity**

Report to the Supervisor's Office and sign in to work with Sally Begay for Tuesday at 0700. Go to the Nurses' Station and find her chart. Open the chart and read the entire Physical & History.

29. For each heading in the left column below, describe the type of data you found in that section of Sally Begay's Physicians' History.

Physicians' History	Type of Data Included
History of present illness	
Family history	
Social history	
Medical history	

Physicians' History	Type of Data Included
Current medications	
Review of systems	

30. Why should a nurse review the Physicians' History?

31. Consider the data documented by the physician in Sally Begay's history. Were any data abnormal or out of the ordinary? In other words, what data suggested possible problem areas for the patient? Record your findings below.

    Data from Physicians' History that are considered out of the ordinary:

32. Close Sally Begay's chart. Now go to her room and conduct a nursing history. Click on **Health History** and systematically go through all the available question areas. Record your data regarding functional health patterns below and on the next two pages.

Note to student: Keep in mind that although the nursing history used at Red Rock Canyon Medical Center is similar to the functional health patterns discussed in your textbook, you will notice some variations. Regardless of the presentation used on the CD, organize your data based on functional health patterns as presented in your textbook.

Nursing History—Functional Health Pattern Data

Health Perception/Health Promotion

Nutritional-Metabolic

Elimination

Nursing History—Functional Health Pattern Data

Activity/Exercise

Sleep-Rest

Cognitive/Perceptual

Self-Perception/Self-Concept

Nursing History—Functional Health Pattern Data

Role/Relationship

Sexuality/Reproductive

Coping/Stress

Value/Belief

33. Consider the data you recorded for question 32. What data did you find out of the ordinary (negative functioning), suggesting a problem or concern? Go back through your data and underline any data you consider to be out of the ordinary.

34. Now compare the data you recorded for question 32 with the functional health patterns history format in your textbook (Table 5-2). What additional questions do you wish the nurse would have asked?

Health History and Physical Examination— Part II

 Reading Assignment: Health History and Physical Examination (Chapter 3)
Patient: Sally Begay, Room 304

This lesson focuses on the physical examination. Perhaps you have covered this content in another course. If so, this lesson will be valuable to you as a review. Begin by reviewing the types and techniques of physical examination.

Writing Activity

1. Several types of physical examinations are listed below. For each type, write a brief description. You may need to refer to other textbooks or sources for help.

Type of Examination	Description
a) Screening examination	
b) Focused examination (also referred to as a "regional" exam)	
c) Comprehensive examination	

Type of Examination	Description
d) Bedside or shift-to-shift examination	

2. Several techniques used during physical examination are listed below and on the next page. For each technique, write a brief description. Refer to your textbook if necessary.

Technique	Description of Technique
Inspection	
Palpation	
Percussion	

Auscultation

CD-ROM Activity

Report to the Supervisor's Office and sign in to work with Sally Begay for the Tuesday 0700 shift. Go to the Nurses' Station and find her chart. Open the chart and browse through the Physical & History.

3. Read the section titled Physical. Referring to the following list of headings, describe the type of data you found in each section of the physical examination.

Physical Examination	Type of Data Included
HEENT	
Cardiopulmonary	
Neurologic	

Physical Examination	Type of Data Included
Musculoskeletal	
Gastrointestinal	
Genitourinary	

4. Consider the data documented by the physician in Sally Begay's physical examination. Were any data abnormal or out of the ordinary? In other words, what data suggested possible problem areas for the patient? Record abnormal findings below.

Data from physician examination that are considered abnormal findings:

5. Based on what you have learned so far, what kinds of cultural issues might become apparent as you perform a physical examination of Sally Begay?

 6. Close Sally Begay's chart. Now go to her room (304) and conduct a physical examination. Click on **Physical** and **Vital Signs** and systematically go through all of the available examination options. As you conduct your examination, do the following three things and record your findings below and on the next two pages.

a. Identify the examination techniques performed by the nurse on the CD.
b. Critique the nurse on the CD. You should notice a few mistakes made in the technique used and/or the documentation done. Can you find them?
c. Record the examination findings.

Area Assessed	What techniques did the nurse use?	What mistakes did you notice in performance or documentation?
Head and Neck		

Area Assessed	What techniques did the nurse use?	What mistakes did you notice in performance or documentation?
Chest/Upper Extremities		
Abdomen and Lower Extremities		

Documentation of Findings

Area Assessed	Findings	
Vital Signs	Temperature: _____	Oxygen saturation: _____
	Heart rate: _____	Blood pressure: _____
	Respiratory rate: _____	Pain rating: _____
Head and Neck		

Area Assessed	What techniques did the nurse use?	What mistakes did you notice in performance or documentation?
Chest/Upper Extremities		
Abdomen and Lower Extremities		

7. Are any of the nursing physical examination data you recorded considered abnormal findings? Go back through your previous findings and underline any abnormal data.

8. Consider data in the nursing history (from Lesson 3) and the nursing physical examination. What should a nurse do with this data once collected?

Patient Teaching

 Reading Assignment: Patient and Family Teaching (Chapter 4)
Patient: Carmen Gonzales, Room 302

You have been assigned to assist with patient teaching for Carmen Gonzales. She is a 56-year-old female admitted to the hospital on Sunday evening through the Emergency Department with a diagnosis of gangrene and osteomyelitis of the left lower leg, diabetes mellitus type 2, and congestive heart failure.

Writing Activity

1. Compare and contrast the two terms *teaching* and *learning* as presented in your textbook. What do these terms actually mean in the context of patient and family teaching?

Teaching

Learning

CD-ROM Activity

Go to the Supervisor's Office and sign in to work with Carmen Gonzales for the Thursday 1100 shift. Then go to one of the computers from which you can access the EPR. Open the EPR for Carmen Gonzales. Next, click on **Admissions** and read the Admissions Profile.

2. Identify significant data from the Admissions Profile that helps you gain an understanding of Carmen Gonzales and her needs from a teaching perspective.

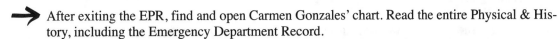 After exiting the EPR, find and open Carmen Gonzales' chart. Read the entire Physical & History, including the Emergency Department Record.

3. Identify significant data from the Emergency Department Record and other sections of the Physical & History that help you gain an understanding of Carmen Gonzales and her needs from a teaching perspective.

 4. Part of developing the overall teaching plan and goals for Carmen Gonzales is dependent on her individual characteristics and her specific health care problems. The textbook identifies several variables to consider, including age, culture, educational level, self-efficacy, and psychologic state. Use your textbook to complete the following exercise.

a. In the second column of the following table, fill in general descriptions of the patient variables listed. You will fill in the third column later.

Patient Variable	Description from Textbook	Application to Carmen Gonzales
Age		
Culture		

Patient Variable	Description from Textbook	Application to Carmen Gonzales
Educational Level		
Self-Efficacy		
Psychologic State		

b. Consider data you previously obtained from the Physicians' History and the Admissions Profile. Use the applicable data to begin filling in the third column of the table above, describing how these variables apply specifically to Carmen Gonzales.

→   c. Now go to Carmen Gonzales' room. Click on **Health History** and collect data. Add any relevant data to the third column of the table.

5. Consider the communication of the nurse conducting the interview with Carmen Gonzales. What behaviors did you observe that were positive communication skills and would facilitate patient teaching?

6. Review the key question list in the following table. Using the data you just collected from the nursing health history, the Physical & History, and the Admissions Profile, indicate which of the key questions for patient teaching assessment have already been addressed. Place an **X** next to those questions where you have sufficient data. Place an **O** next to those areas where additional assessment still needs to be conducted.

Table 5-1 Assessment of Characteristics That Affect Patient Teaching

Characteristic		Key Questions
Readiness to learn	___	What has your physician or nurse practitioner told you about your health problem?
	___	What behaviors could make your problem better or worse?
Biophysical	___	What is the primary diagnosis?
	___	Are there additional diagnoses?
	___	Is the patient acutely ill?
	___	How old is the patient?
	___	What is the patient's current mental status?
	___	What is the patient's hearing ability? Visual ability? Motor ability?
	___	Is the patient fatigued? In pain?
	___	What medications is the patient on? How might these affect learning?
Psychologic	___	Does the patient appear anxious? Afraid? Depressed? Defensive?
	___	Is the patient in a state of denial?
Sociocultural	___	Does the patient have family or close friends?
	___	What is the patient's belief regarding his or her illness or treatment?
	___	Is the proposed change consistent with the patient's cultural values?
Socioeconomic	___	Does the patient work?
	___	What is the patient's occupation?
	___	What is the patient's living arrangement?
Learning style	___	Does the patient "learn best" through visual (reading), auditory (tape or lecture), or physical stimuli (demonstration)?
	___	In what kind of environment does the patient learn best? Formal classroom? Informal setting, such as home or office? Alone or among peers? What prior learning experiences were helpful?

→ Go to the Nurses' Station and find the location of the health team meeting for Carmen Gonzales. Attend the meeting, listening carefully to the suggestions of the three individuals. If desired, go back to the patient's chart, click on **Health Team**, and read the written reports.

7. Below and on the following page, record some of the key issues the clinical nurse specialist, nurse case manager, and social worker have identified regarding Carmen Gonzales' discharge planning.

Discharge Planning Team Report—Student Notes

Health Team Member	Key Issues from Report
Rose Simpson, Case Manager	

Health Team Member	Key Issues from Report
Louise Johnson, CNS	
Kris Holmes, MSW	

8. Considering everything you currently know about Carmen Gonzales, make a list of *at least* five different things you could potentially teach this patient to enhance her care once she goes home.

9. Choose one of the patient teaching needs from your list in question 8. In the space below, address some of the issues that would be central to your teaching strategy.

Issue	How will you deal with this?
Communication	
Method of Teaching	
Involvement of Patient and Family	

6

Complementary and Alternative Therapies

/O⃝⊘ **Reading Assignment:** Complementary and Alternative Therapies (Chapter 7)
Patients: Carmen Gonzales, Room 302
David Ruskin, Room 303
Sally Begay, Room 304
Ira Bradley, Room 309
Andrea Wang, Room 310

This lesson focuses on the possible application of various complementary and alternative therapies for the patients in Red Rock Canyon Medical Center. For this lesson, you will not need to use your *Virtual Clinical Excursions* CD.

 Before you begin, review some of the basic concepts presented in your textbook regarding complementary and alternative therapies.

 Writing Activity

Indicate whether the following statements regarding complementary or alternative therapies are true or false.

1. _____ Complementary or alternative therapies are less effective than conventional allopathic/Western approaches to health care.

2. _____ Complementary or alternative therapies may be considered "conventional" in other countries.

3. _____ Approximately 75% of people in the United States rely on one or more forms of complementary or alternative therapies.

4. _____ Worldwide, the United States has been the leader in the development and the acceptance of complementary or alternative therapies.

5. _____ Many complementary and alternative therapies are consistent with many values within the domain of nursing.

6. What are the two primary goals of the National Center for Complementary and Alternative Medicine (NCCAM)?

 Match each of the following descriptions with the corresponding complementary or alternative therapy, and identify the NCCAM category to which it belongs. Use your textbook for help.

Description

Complementary and Alternative Therapy

7. _____/_____ Dietary modification that includes the elimination of meat, animal fat, eggs, poultry, dairy products, simple sugars, and artificially produced foods in the diet

8. _____/_____ Facilitates the expression of emotions, memories, and concerns through artistic methods

9. _____/_____ Treatment involves the manipulation of the spinal column; based on the theory that state of health is determined by condition of the nervous system

10. _____/_____ Focuses on restoring and maintaining the balanced flow of vital energy, using a variety of interventions, including acupuncture, Tai Chi, herbology, diet, and meditation

11. _____/_____ The use of hands to direct or modulate human energy fields to improve sense of well-being and reduce sense of stress and discomfort

12. _____/_____ Ancient system of exercise that focuses on creating balance and enhancing self-regulation in the body

13. _____/_____ Manipulation of soft tissue through stroking, rubbing, or kneading to increase circulation, improve muscle tone, and produce relaxation

14. _____/_____ Topical application or inhalation of essential oils (from plant extracts) to promote and maintain overall health

15. _____/_____ A system originating in India that focuses on the balance of mind, body, and spirit; interventions include diet, detoxification, breathing exercises, meditation, and yoga

16. _____/_____ A self-directed practice of focusing, centering, and relaxing the mind and body; used to reduce stress and to promote health

17. _____/_____ Use of magnets and magnetic energy to improve blood flow and reduce pain

18. _____/_____ An approach developed in the United States that emphasizes restoration and maintenance of overall health as opposed to symptoms

a. Aromatherapy
b. Art therapy
c. Ayurveda
d. Chiropractic therapy
e. Macrobiotic diet
f. Meditation
g. Magnetic therapy
h. Naturopathy
i. Therapeutic massage
j. Therapeutic touch
k. Traditional Chinese medicine
l. Qigong

NCCAM Category

- Alternative Medical Systems (**AMS**)
- Mind-Body Interventions (**MBI**)
- Biologic-Based Therapies (**BBT**)
- Manipulative and Body-Based Methods (**MBBM**)
- Energy Therapies (**ET**)

Now consider the application of these various complementary therapies to each of the patients in Red Rock Canyon Medical Center.

19. Below and on the next four pages, you will find a brief summary of data for each patient. Based on this data, circle the complementary therapies that are most likely to be accepted by the patient and might be helpful to the patient if offered. Justify your answers in the right-hand column.

Patient Data	Complementary Therapies	Justification for or Against Use
Carmen Gonzales **Room 302** **56-year-old female** **Dx:** Diabetes mellitus type 2, CHF, osteomyelitis **Cultural group:** Hispanic-American **Primary issues:** • Having a great deal of pain in the leg from the foot infection • Has lack of understanding of medications, diet, and disease processes • Very anxious about going home and managing care • Insufficient social and financial support **Other data:** • Is Catholic—indicated an interest in having a priest visit her	Chiropractic therapy Spirituality Meditation Traditional Chinese medicine Relaxation Imagery Acupuncture Therapeutic touch Biofeedback Massage therapy Herbal therapy	

Patient Data	Complementary Therapies	Justification for or Against Use
David Ruskin **Room 303** **31-year-old male**	Chiropractic therapy	
Dx: Bike accident—CHI and fractured humerus **Cultural:** African-American **Primary issues:** • Having a great deal of pain in the arm and headaches • Initially had some confusion from CHI • Concerns about regaining independence and athletic training schedule	Spirituality Meditation Traditional Chinese medicine	
Other data: • Very interested in diet and exercise and maintaining high level of health • Describes self as spiritual, but not religious • Well-educated man— finishing master's degree • Good social and financial support	Relaxation Imagery Acupuncture Therapeutic touch Biofeedback Massage therapy Herbal therapy	

Patient Data	Complementary Therapies	Justification for or Against Use
Sally Begay **Room 304** **58-year-old female**	Chiropractic therapy	
Dx: Bacterial pneumonia, chronic bronchitis, hypertension **Cultural:** Traditional Navajo **Primary issues:**	Spirituality	
• Has problems with shortness of breath and fatigue • Is concerned about keeping up with work on farm at home	Meditation	
• Lives in rural setting miles from primary health care provider; access to health care is concern	Traditional Chinese medicine	
• Lives in rural area; is in need of educational outreach to prevent further infections	Relaxation	
• Need to provide culturally sensitive care	Imagery	
Other data: • Cultural practices important to her are medicine man and regular doctor	Acupuncture	
• Recently had healing ceremony done for her and will have another one when she gets home	Therapeutic touch	
• Good social support	Biofeedback	
	Massage therapy	
	Herbal therapy	

Patient Data	Complementary Therapies	Justification for or Against Use
Ira Bradley **Room 309** **43-year-old male**	Chiropractic therapy	
Dx: Late-stage HIV, *Pneumocystis carinii* pneumonia, candidiasis, Kaposi's sarcoma **Cultural:** American Jewish	Spirituality	
Primary issues: • Pain/discomfort • Nutrition • Oral mucosa	Meditation	
• Chronic fatigue • Depression (knows he is dying) • Ineffective family coping	Traditional Chinese medicine	
• Lack of adequate financial and social support	Relaxation	
Other data: • Sees psychotherapist for depression • Does not want hospital chaplain, but would appreciate visit from rabbi	Imagery	
	Acupuncture	
	Therapeutic touch	
	Biofeedback	
	Massage therapy	
	Herbal therapy	

Patient Data	Complementary Therapies	Justification for or Against Use
Andrea Wang **Room 310** **20-year-old female**	Chiropractic therapy	
Dx: Acute spinal cord injury; paralysis **Cultural:** Chinese-American **Primary issues:** • Paralysis—paraplegia • Regaining independence • Resuming relationship with boyfriend • Sexuality • Resuming education/career goals • Concern regarding care for parents • Ineffective family coping • Possible lack of adequate social support **Other data:** • Is a first-generation Chinese-American; primarily has Western values; however, some Chinese traditions practiced at home (mainly by parents)	Spirituality Meditation Traditional Chinese medicine Relaxation Imagery Acupuncture Therapeutic touch Biofeedback Massage therapy Herbal therapy	

20. In the previous activity, you were limited to the listed choices of complementary therapies. Now you are encouraged to consider other therapies that each of these patients might benefit from. Below, list additional complementary therapies discussed in your textbook that might be appropriate to offer to these patients.

Patient	Additional Therapies	Justification
Carmen Gonzales		
David Ruskin		
Sally Begay		
Ira Bradley		
Andrea Wang		

LESSON 7

Stress Response

 Reading Assignment: Stress (Chapter 8)
Patient: David Ruskin, Room 303

This lesson focuses on the response to physical and psychologic stress. You will conduct an analysis and application of the stress response by considering the effect of stress on one of the Red Rock Canyon Medical Center patients, David Ruskin.

 Begin by reviewing the three theories of stress presented in your textbook. Match each of the following theories with the corresponding description.

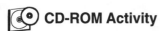 **Writing Activity**

Stress Theory	Description
1. _____ Stress as a stimulus	a. A particular relationship between the person and the environment that taxes or exceeds his or her resources.
2. _____ Stress as a transaction	
3. _____ Stress as a response (general adaptation syndrome)	b. A nonspecific response of the body to any demand made on it, physical or psychologic.
	c. An event that causes a response; frequent life changes make individuals more vulnerable to illness.

CD-ROM Activity

Go to the Supervisor's Office and sign in to work with David Ruskin on Tuesday at 0700. To find out what happened to this patient, go to the Nurses' Station and open his chart. Read the Physical & History, including the Emergency Department Report. Then click on **Nurses' Notes**. Read the nurses' notes for Sunday and Monday.

4. List the physical stressors David Ruskin experienced on Sunday.

The physiologic response to stress is initiated with the processing of the stressful stimuli by the cerebral cortex. The hypothalamus essentially triggers activation in the sympathetic nervous system, and stimulation of the anterior and posterior pituitary glands. Match each of the following physical responses with the corresponding triggering event. (Answers will be used more than once. Refer to your textbook for help if necessary.)

Physical Response	**Triggering Event**
5. _____ Increased ADH secretion	a. Stimulation of sympathetic activity
6. _____ Increased epinephrine	
7. _____ Increased blood glucose	b. Stimulation of anterior pituitary gland hormone
8. _____ Decreased peristalsis	
9. _____ Increased aldosterone secretion	c. Stimulation of posterior pituitary gland
10. _____ Decreased immune response	
11. _____ Increased cardiac output	
12. _____ Dilation of vessels in skeletal muscles	
13. _____ Decreased allergic response	
14. _____ Increased norepinephrine secretion	

15. For each of the following vital signs or body functions, indicate what you guess David Ruskin's physical reaction was during the time immediately following the accident. Mark with ↑ or ↓, unless otherwise indicated.

___ Blood pressure   ____ Gastrointestinal motility

___ Heart rate   ____ Perspiration

___ Respiratory rate   ____ Pupils (**Constriction** or **Dilation**)

16. Note David Ruskin's admitting vital signs documented in the Emergency Department. Record them in the spaces provided.

Temperature _____ Heart rate _____ Respiration _____ Blood pressure _____

17. Based on his vital signs at the time of Emergency Department evaluation, which stage would you guess David Ruskin was experiencing? (Circle the stage.)

Stage of alarm

Stage of resistance

Stage of exhaustion

→ 18. Consider David Ruskin's condition now—Tuesday morning, 2 days post-injury. Conduct a nursing assessment of the patient's stress and his ability to cope with it. In the space below, identify current possible sources of David Ruskin's stress. Then identify factors in his life that help him resist stress (see your textbook for factors that affect an individual's response to stress). Use data from the following three sources to complete your assessment:

- Chart: Physical & History
- EPR: Admissions Profile
- Inside David Ruskin's room:
  - Click on **Health History**; collect data from the nursing history.
  - Click on **Vital Signs**, then **Pain Rating**.

Current Possible Sources of Stress	Factors That Help to Resist Stress

19. The nurse should assess not only for stressors the patient may be experiencing but also for adequate coping measures. Below is a list of coping resources discussed in the textbook. Circle all that seem to apply to David Ruskin based on the data you have collected.

Robust health	Communication skills	Self-efficacy
High energy level	Collection of information	Spiritual faith
High morale	Social networks	Adequate finances

20. Based on your assessment of David Ruskin's stressors, factors that help him resist stress, and coping measures, what specific nursing interventions can you think of that will assist this patient further in managing the stress he is currently experiencing?

 21. What is your overall evaluation of how David Ruskin is currently handling his stress? Does he seem to be managing it well? Do you have any areas of concern that could prove to be problematic? Which, if any, of the nursing diagnoses listed in Table 8-8 of your textbook are applicable to David Ruskin?

LESSON 8

Pain

/OℛᎧ **Reading Assignment:** Nursing Management: Pain (Chapter 9)
Patients: David Ruskin, Room 303
        Ira Bradley, Room 309

In this activity, you will compare the pain experience of two different patients—from assessment to management. To do this, you will complete a pain assessment tool on the following two patients:
- David Ruskin, a 31-year-old male patient who was hit by a car while riding his bike. This patient has many injuries, including a closed head injury, a fracture to the right arm, and a chest contusion.
- Ira Bradley, a 43-year-old male who was admitted to the hospital with late-stage HIV, *Pneumocystis carinii* pneumonia, candidiasis and Kaposi's sarcoma.

CD-ROM Activity

1. Review the pain assessment tool on the following page. Complete a pain assessment tool for David Ruskin and Ira Bradley based on data you collect from various parts of the charts as well from each patient. (*Note: you may not find all the information you need to complete the tool.*) Specifically, you should do all of the following for each patient:

- Go to the Supervisor's Office and sign in to work with the patient on Tuesday at 0700.

- Proceed to the Nurses' Station and open the patient's chart. Read the Physical & History, including the Emergency Room Report.

- Click on the **Nurses' Notes** and read the notes from Sunday until present.

- Click on **Expired MARs**. Determine the following: What pain medication has the patient received since admission? What dose has the patient received? How often has the medication been given?

- Close the chart and open the patient's EPR. Click on **Vital Signs** and review the previous pain assessment for the patient since admission.

- Close the EPR and open the MAR. What medications are available to the patient today for pain?

- Close the MAR and go into the patient's room. Click on **Vital Signs**, then **Pain Assessment**. Listen to the patient describe the pain. Click on **Continue Working with Patient**, then on **Medications** to see what medications the nurse is preparing to give. Finally, click on **Health History** and select various questions to collect data. Note any data that might be helpful in explaining the pain experience for the patient.

83

Pain Assessment Tool—David Ruskin
Tuesday 0800

Etiology (disease process and physical findings associated with pain) _____

_____

Type of Pain (circle one) ⟶ acute   chronic nonmalignant   malignant

Location of Pain (indicate location of pain using figure in box)

Right   Left   Left   Right

Description of the Pain Pattern

Pain Intensity

0 1 2 3 4 5 6 7 8 9 10

Description of the Pain Quality

Variables Affecting the Pain Experience

Affective

Behavioral

Cognitive

Record of Pain Medications Given and Effectiveness

Day	Medication, Dose, and Time Given	Effectiveness
Sunday		
Monday		
Tuesday		

Pain Assessment Tool—Ira Bradley
Tuesday 0800

Etiology (disease process and physical findings associated with pain) _____

_____

Type of Pain (circle one) ⟶ acute   chronic nonmalignant   malignant

Location of Pain (indicate location of pain using figure in box)

Description of the Pain Pattern

Pain Intensity

0 1 2 3 4 5 6 7 8 9 10

Description of the Pain Quality

Variables Affecting the Pain Experience

Affective

Behavioral

Cognitive

Record of Pain Medications Given and Effectiveness

Day	Medication, Dose, and Time Given	Effectiveness
Sunday		
Monday		
Tuesday		

2. What additional data would have been helpful to complete the pain assessment tool? In the space below, write additional questions you would have asked either patient or identify data you think should have been on the chart.

3. Compare the data on the two pain assessment tools. What similarities do you see? What differences are there?

Similarities   **Differences**

4. How do the terms *mild pain*, *moderate pain*, and *severe pain* correlate to the pain intensity scale?

5. How should the pain intensity scale ratings given by the two patients be interpreted? (Circle one for each patient.)

   David Ruskin: mild pain   moderate pain   severe pain

   Ira Bradley: mild pain   moderate pain   severe pain

6. Only one of the patients was medicated for pain on Tuesday morning. Which patient was medicated for pain? Should both have received pain medication? Why or why not? Can you think of reasons one of the patients did not receive pain medications?

7. Analgesic medications are grouped as Step 1, Step 2 and Step 3 on the analgesic ladder. To what do these levels refer?

Step	Type of Pain	Type of Analgesics Used
1		
2		
3		

8. Consider the pain medications ordered for each patient. Were the medications consistent with the type of pain the patient was experiencing? What recommendations might you make regarding analgesia for these patients?

9. What additional nonpharmacologic pain relief strategies would be appropriate for you, as a student nurse, to offer to Ira Bradley and David Ruskin?

Patient	Nonpharmacologic Strategies
David Ruskin	
Ira Bradley	

10. Before you walk into David Ruskin's room, you hear him laughing. When you enter, you see that he has visitors from the university. When you ask him to rate his pain, he tells you his pain is 8/10. What should you record?
    a. "Pain rating 8/10."
    b. "Pain rating 7/10."
    c. "Pain rating 6/10."
    d. "Patient states 8/10, but this is probably not accurate rating."

11. If you administer to David Ruskin oxycodone hydrochloride 5 to 10 mg PO (immediate release) at 0800, approximately what time would it reach peak effect?
    a. 0815
    b. 0830
    c. 0900
    d. 1000

12. Ira Bradley has a pain rating of 9/10. What medication should be offered to him?
    a. Morphine 2 to 8 mg IV
    b. Morphine 30 mg PO
    c. Tylenol 600 mg PO
    d. Oxycodone 10 mg PO

13. Ira Bradley is not sure he wants pain medication because he is concerned about addiction. Which of the following responses by the nurse would be best in this situation?
    a. "I am glad you are concerned about this. Let me know when you really need the medication."
    b. "Since your condition is terminal, addiction is the last thing you should be concerned about."
    c. "Although you may become addicted, we have medications available to help you overcome the addiction."
    d. "Addiction is a common concern patients have, but the truth is, less than 0.1% of people who take pain medication for medical therapy become addicted."

LESSON 9 ————————————————————

Inflammation and Infection

 Reading Assignment: Nursing Management: Inflammation, Infection, and Healing
(Chapter 12)
Patient: Carmen Gonzales, Room 302

Carmen Gonzales was admitted to the hospital on Sunday with a gangrene infection and osteomyelitis to the lower left leg. In the following activities, you will apply the concepts of infection and inflammation as you consider nursing care for this patient.

Writing Activity

1. Before you begin, answer the following general question: How does a bacterial infection cause lethal cell injury?

CD-ROM Activity

Go to the Supervisor's Office and sign in to work with Carmen Gonzales on Tuesday at 0700. Proceed to the Nurses' Station and open the patient's chart. Read the Physical & History section, including the Emergency Room Record, and answer the following questions.

2. Besides gangrene and osteomyelitis, what other three medical diagnoses are identified upon admission?

a.

b.

c.

3. What are Carmen Gonzales' symptoms upon presentation to the Emergency Department?

4. What are her vital signs at admission?

   Temperature _____ Heart rate _____ Respiratory rate _____ Blood pressure _____

5. What is the relationship between the leg infection and the clinical findings? How can these findings be explained? Below and on the next page, explain the cause and meaning of each of the findings listed.

Clinical Findings	Cause and Meaning of Findings
Fever	
Increased heart rate and respiratory rate	
Malaise, nausea, and anorexia	

Clinical Findings	**Cause and Meaning of Findings**
Pain in the leg	

6. In the Emergency Department Record, the physician describes an area of necrosis on the medial side of her left leg. What does the term *necrosis* mean?

 7. What is a common cause of gangrenous necrosis? (Refer to Table 12-4 in your textbook.) Is there any correlation between Carmen Gonzales' other medical problems and the development of gangrenous necrosis? If so, what might that correlation be?

→ Now click on **Physicians' Orders**. Read the orders for Sunday at 1830.

8. The physician ordered a complete blood count (CBC) and a wound culture on Sunday at 1830. What is the rationale for these tests?

9. Note this order on Sunday evening: "Op permit for surgical debridement . . . ." What is a surgical debridement? Why is the physician going to do this?

10. Find a physician order for wound care in post-op orders on Monday. Record that wound care order below.

11. What is your opinion regarding the dressing change order? What additional information would you expect? What seems to be missing?

12. Close the chart. Go to the computer under the bookshelf and open the EPR for Carmen Gonzales. Click on **Hematology** and record the CBC and differential results for Sunday evening below.

Lab Test	Result	Lab Test	Result
Hgb		Neutrophil segs %	
Hct		Neutrophil bands %	
RBC		Lymphocytes %	
Platelets		Monocytes %	
WBC		Eosinophils %	
		Basophils %	

Which of the results are abnormal? Circle each abnormal result and indicate whether it is high or low. What is your interpretation of the CBC results? Do any of these results surprise you? (Refer to Appendix B in your textbook for help.)

→ Close the EPR. Now go to the blue notebook on the counter and open the MAR for Carmen Gonzales.

13. What medication is being given on Tuesday for Carmen Gonzales' infection? Fill in the missing data in the medication order below.

_____   _____ grams   IVPB   q _____ hours
    (name of medication)   (dose)   (route)   (frequency)

Times the medication is due on Tuesday: _____   _____   _____   _____

14. What other two medications can the nurse administer to help treat symptoms associated with the inflammatory process? When should they be given?

Medication and Dose	Given for What Reason? How often?
Acetaminophen 650 mg PO	
Morphine 2 to 5 mg IM	
Oxycodone 10 mg PO	

15. Before you administer a medication, you must be familiar with that agent. Fill out the following drug card for cefoxitin. (You will probably need to refer to your nursing drug book.)

Cefoxitin Drug Card

Classification:

Action:

Indications:

Contraindications/Precautions:

Major Adverse Effects:

Typical Dose:

IV Administration:

---

16. Close the MAR. Consider the nursing interventions discussed in the textbook. Nursing interventions include fever management, administration of antibiotics to treat the infection, wound management, and pain management. What other nursing measures should be included in your plan of care for Carmen Gonzales? Provide a rationale for each of your planned measures.

Nursing Measure   **Rationale**

17. Refer to Carmen Gonzales' CBC differential count results you recorded earlier in this lesson. Which of the following explains why the eosinophils are not elevated?
    a. Eosinophils are chronically low in patients with diabetes.
    b. An increase in eosinophils is usually associated with allergic reaction.
    c. Eosinophils are never elevated in the presence of anemia.
    d. An increase in neutrophils causes phagocytosis of eosinophils.

18. Carmen Gonzales had purulent drainage from her wound infection. Which of the following describes the cause of exudate formation?
    a. Cellular lysis from bacterial invasion and destruction
    b. Fluid and leukocytes move to the site of infection
    c. Cellular release of histamine
    d. Fluid shift from intracellular to extracelluar space

19. It is 0700 on Tuesday morning. Carmen Gonzales' vital signs are as follows: Temp 102.6° F, HR 108, RR 22, and BP 138/88. Which of the following nursing measures is most appropriate in response to this data?
    a. Elevate the patient's left leg.
    b. Change the dressing on the wound.
    c. Administer the antibiotic cefoxitin now.
    d. Administer acetaminophen now.

20. The nurse anticipates that Carmen Gonzales may experience delayed wound healing for which of the following reasons?
    a. She has diabetes.
    b. She had a surgical debridement.
    c. She had a lot of pain in the leg.
    d. She had an elevated WBC.

21. In order to reduce the spread of infection to this patient, which of the following nursing measures, in addition to handwashing, should be followed?
    a. Wear eye protection and a mask (or face shield) during dressing changes.
    b. Use sterile linens when making the patient's bed.
    c. Follow meticulous aseptic technique during dressing changes to her leg.
    d. Place the patient in protective isolation.

HIV—Part I

👓 **Reading Assignment:** Nursing Management: Human Immunodeficiency Virus
Infection (Chapter 14)

Patient: Ira Bradley, Room 309

You have been assigned to care for Ira Bradley, a 41-year-old man admitted to the hospital on
Sunday with late-stage HIV, *Pneumocystis carinii* pneumonia, candidiasis, and Kaposi's sarcoma. In order to provide competent care, you must first prepare by reading his chart and considering care as outlined in your textbook.

 CD-ROM Activity

Go to the Supervisor's Office and sign in to work with Ira Bradley for the Tuesday 0700 shift.
Proceed to the Nurses' Station and open the patient's chart. Read the Physical & History, includ-
ing the Emergency Department Report. Click on **Physicians' Orders** and read the orders for
Sunday. Answer the following questions, based on what you have read.

✏️ **Writing Activity**

1. Ira Bradley has had an HIV infection for several years. What was the primary reason his
wife brought him to the hospital on Sunday?

2. Based on data in the chart, circle the HIV infection phase below that is consistent with Ira Bradley's condition. Provide a rationale based on criteria found in your textbook.

HIV Infection Phase	Rationale
Acute retroviral syndrome	
Early infection (asymptomatic)	
Early symptomatic disease	
AIDS	

3. According to the Emergency Department Report, the physician suspected several opportunistic infections and diseases. For each of these conditions, compare Ira Bradley's situation (according to the ER records and initial admission orders) with textbook descriptions in the following three areas: clinical findings, diagnostic tests, and treatment initiated. (Refer to Table 14-2 in the textbook for help.)

Opportunistic Disease/Infection	Clinical Findings	
	Typical Findings According to Textbook	Ira Bradley's Findings
Pneumocystis carinii pneumonia		
Kaposi's sarcoma		
Candida (oral candidiasis)		

Opportunistic Disease/Infection	Diagnostic Tests	
	Typical Tests According to Textbook	Ira Bradley's Tests
Pneumocystis carinii pneumonia		
Kaposi's sarcoma		
Candida (oral candidiasis)		

Opportunistic Disease/Infection	Treatment (Medications)	
	Typical Treatment According to Textbook	Ira Bradley's Treatment
Pneumocystis carinii pneumonia		
Kaposi's sarcoma		
Candida (oral candidiasis)		

4. Consider the figure below showing a timeline spectrum of HIV infection. How does Ira Bradley's condition compare with this figure based on what you know?

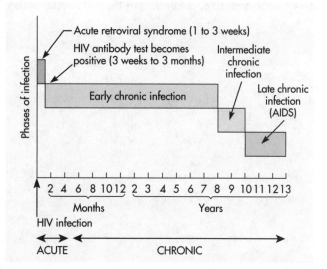

Now click on **Nurses' Notes** in Ira Bradley's chart. Read the notes for Sunday, Monday, and Tuesday morning.

5. What pattern of change is noted over the last few shifts?

→ Close the chart. Click on the computer below the bookshelf and open Ira Bradley's EPR.

6. Review the vital signs taken since admission. What sorts of patterns do you see in Ira Bradley's vital signs over the course of the last couple of days?

7. Review the pain assessment since admission. What sorts of patterns do you see in Ira Bradley's level and type of pain over the course of the last couple of days?

8. Check Ira Bradley's CBC and chemistry lab results from Sunday night. Record the results below and on the next page. Circle any abnormal findings and indicate whether the result is higher or lower than normal range. In the right-hand column, indicate the significance of any of these findings. The first one is done for you.

Lab Test	Result	What does it reflect?
Sodium	152 (high)	Hypernatremia consistent with dehydration
Potassium		
Chloride		
CO_2		
BUN		
Creatinine		
Albumin		
Hemoglobin		

Lab Test	Result	What does it reflect?
Hematocrit		
RBCs		
Platelets		

➤ Close the EPR. Now go to the MAR and open Ira Bradley's record. Review the routine medications he is receiving.

9. Using your textbook and a drug reference, determine the classification of each drug ordered for Ira Bradley (listed below and on the next page) and provide a reason that the drug has been ordered. Check to verify that the dosage and route are within recommended guidelines.

Medication, Dose, Route	Classification	Reason Ordered
D_5 0.45 NS @ 125 cc/hour		
AZT 1 mg/kg IVPB over 1h, q4h x 24 doses		
Trimethoprim 300 mg and sulfamethoxazole 1.5 g IVPB q6h x 16 doses		

Medication, Dose, Route	Classification	Reason Ordered
Delavirdine myselate 400 mg PO TID		
Saquinovir 1200 mg PO TID within 2h of eating		
Fluconazole 100 mg PO in A.M. x 14 days		
Alitretinoin gel 0.1%, apply to lesions, BID		
Hydroxyurea		

10. Why are three antiretroviral agents included in the routine medications given to Ira Bradley? What is the advantage of administering three as opposed to just one?

11. Consider Ira Bradley's condition and physician orders. What type of precautions must the nurse take to prevent spread of HIV to himself or herself, as well as to other patients? What infection control concerns should the nurse have on behalf of Ira Bradley?

12. When Ira Bradley arrived to the Emergency Department on Sunday, the nurse recorded the following vital signs: Temp 100.1° F, BP 105/75, RR 23, HR 95, O_2 sat 85% on room air. Based on these findings, which of the following interventions should the nurse take immediately?
   a. Administer acetaminophen for the fever.
   b. Place Ira Bradley in the supine position with his legs elevated.
   c. Start an IV line.
   d. Administer oxygen.

13. Which of the following laboratory tests is frequently used to evaluate the status and guide treatment of a patient with HIV infection but has not been ordered for Ira Bradley?
   a. CD4+ T cell count
   b. Blood cultures
   c. Lung tissue biopsy
   d. Stool culture

14. Ira Bradley was in the hospital 6 weeks ago for *Pneumocystis carinii* pneumonia. This fact supports which of the following statements?
   a. He has not been compliant with his medication regime.
   b. The infection from 6 weeks ago has now spread to his mouth.
   c. The HIV agents he is taking are not effective.
   d. These infections tend to be cyclical because they usually are not fully eradicated.

15. The initial disorientation Ira Bradley experienced during the first few days of hospitalization can best be explained by:
   a. cryptococcal meningitis.
   b. closed head injury from the fall.
   c. fluid and electrolyte imbalances.
   d. side effects of antiretroviral therapy.

16. At this point in time, which of the following focuses of care seem to be most applicable?
   a. Patient and family teaching regarding prevention of HIV transmission (e.g., using sterile linens when making the patient's bed)
   b. Identification of social and financial support for the patient and family
   c. Discussion with patient and family regarding progress in the development of the HIV vaccine
   d. Discussion with the family regarding the possible use of restraints

HIV—Part II

Reading Assignment: Nursing Management: Human Immunodeficiency Virus
Infection (Chapter 14)
Patient: Ira Bradley, Room 309

In this lesson, you will continue to care for Ira Bradley, a 41-year-old man admitted to the hospital on Sunday with late-stage HIV, *Pneumocystis carinii* pneumonia, candidiasis, and Kaposi's sarcoma. In Lesson 10, you prepared by reading his chart and considering his care as outlined in your textbook. In this lesson, you will participate in the patient's care.

 CD-ROM Activity

Go to the Supervisor's Office and sign in to work with Ira Bradley for the Tuesday 0700 shift. Proceed to the Nurses' Station and check the bulletin board to determine where report is being given for this patient. Go to that location and listen to the report.

Writing Activity

1. As you listen to the report on Ira Bradley, record pertinent information using the form on the following page.

Red Rock Canyon Medical Center
Report Notes

Patient: _____ Room # _____

Age: _____ Diagnosis: _____

Vital signs: _____ O_2 sat:_____ Pain: _____

Treatments:

Significant assessment findings:

IV location/date: _____

Identified patient/family problems:

2. What did you think of the report? What information was not given by the nurse that you think should have been included? What information were you given that you did not find helpful?

3. It is now 0730. Go to the MAR in the Nurses' Station. Click open Ira Bradley's MAR and identify the medications you will need to give him this morning. For each of the medications listed below, record the times that drug is due today between 0800 and 1500.

Routine medications, dose, and route	Time due	PRN medications given since midnight last night (including dose and time given)
AZT 1 mg/kg IVPB over 1 hour, q4h x 24 doses		
Trimethoprim 300 mg and sulfamethoxazole 1.5 g IVPB q6h x 16 doses		
Delavirdine myselate 400 mg PO TID		
Saquinovir 1200 mg PO TID within 2 hours of eating		
Fluconazole 100 mg PO A.M. x 14 days		
Alitretinoin gel 0.1%, apply to lesions BID		

4. It is now 0800. The primary nurse tells you she will take care of the 0800 medications while you obtain a set of vital signs. Go into Ira Bradley's room and click on **Vital Signs**. Obtain a full set of vital signs and record them below.

Blood pressure _____   Heart rate _____

Respiration _____   Temperature _____

Oxygen saturation _____   Pain location _____

Pain characteristics _____   Level of pain   1 2 3 4 5 6 7 8 9 10

5. Is Ira Bradley wearing oxygen at the time the oxygen saturation is taken?

6. Is the use of oxygen significant when documenting oxygen saturation levels? Why or why not? What should be recorded when documenting oxygen saturation?

7. Based on the vital signs, write the appropriate three-part nursing diagnosis evident at this time and some appropriate nursing interventions.

Nursing Diagnosis   **Interventions**

_____

related to _____

_____

_____

as manifested by _____

_____

_____

8. It is now 0830—time to conduct your bedside nursing assessment. Click on **Physical Assessment** and obtain data from the physical examination. Record your findings below and on the next page. Circle any findings that are considered abnormal.

Examination   **Findings**

Head and Neck

Examination	Findings

Chest/
Upper Extremities

Abdomen and
Lower Extremities

9. Based on the data you heard in report earlier this morning, there are a couple of other things the nurse should have included during the examination—one involving the upper extremities and one involving the lower extremities. What is missing?

Upper extremities

Lower extremities

➡ It is 0900—time to give medications. While in Ira Bradley's room, click on **Medications**. Now click on **Review Medications**, and a pop-up box will appear, listing medications the nurse is preparing to administer. Next, click on **Administer**, and you will see the nurse giving him his medications.

10. a. Which medication is the nursing giving 1 hour later than indicated on the MAR?

b. Is this a serious issue? Why or why not?

c. How should this be documented on the MAR?

d. What further action by the nurse is appropriate?

11. a. What medication is due at 0900 but does not appear on the pop-up box while the nurse is administering medications?

   b. Where is a medication like this frequently kept?

   c. What is a likely explanation for not seeing this medication given at this time?

12. It is now 1000. While still in Ira Bradley's room, click on **Health History**. Record significant data below and on the next two pages.

Area	Data
Perception/ Self-Concept	
Activity	

Area	Data
Sexuality/Reproduction	
Culture	
Nutrition/Metabolic	
Sleep/Rest	

Area	Data
Role/Relationship	
Health Perception	
Elimination	
Cognitive/Perceptual	

Area	Data
Coping/Stress	
Values/Beliefs	

 13. Review ongoing care in the Ambulatory and Home Care section in your textbook. How are the concepts presented in these sections relevant to Ira Bradley?

14. Based on your interview, examination findings, and information from the chart, develop a list of nursing diagnoses and collaborative problems for Ira Bradley. Be sure you can support all of the problems you select with data. Use your textbook for additional help.

Nursing Diagnoses   **Collaborative Problems**

15. From the problem list you developed in question 14, choose two problems and develop them further. For each problem, identify patient outcomes and nursing interventions specific for Ira Bradley. Why did you select the ones that you did?

Nursing Diagnosis or Collaborative Problem	Outcomes	Nursing Interventions

Cancer

 Reading Assignment: Cancer (Chapter 15)
Patient: Ira Bradley, Room 309

Once again, you have been assigned to care for Ira Bradley. Remember that he is a 43-year-old man admitted to the hospital on Sunday with late-stage HIV, *Pneumocystis carinii* pneumonia, candidiasis, and Kaposi's sarcoma.

Before you begin working with Ira Bradley, review a few concepts associated with cancer.

Writing Activity

1. Briefly describe what is meant by the following three stages in the development of cancer.

Cancer Stage	Description
Initiation	
Promotion	

Cancer Stage	Description
Progression	

2. The textbook describes the immune system role in the recognition and destruction of tumor cells. Briefly describe the response to tumor-associated antigens (TAAs) by immunologic surveillance.

3. Briefly describe the following four specific immune responses to tumor cells.

Immune Response	Description
Cytotoxic T cells	
Natural killer cells (NK)	

Immune Response	Description
Macrophages	
B-lymphocytes	

4. One of Ira Bradley's admitting diagnoses is Kaposi's sarcoma (KS) on the left leg. What is KS?

CD-ROM Activity

Go to the Supervisor's Office and sign in to work with Ira Bradley for the Tuesday 0700 shift. Your first task is to collect data. Specifically, you are interested in data associated with KS. Proceed to the Nurses' Station and open Ira Bradley's EPR. Read his Admissions Profile, taking notes as you read.

5. What information is found in the profile related to KS?

Notes from Admissions Profile

Close the EPR and open Ira Bradley's chart. Read the Physical & History, including the Emergency Department Report.

6. What mention is made of KS in the Physical & History? Is there any indication of current or recent past treatment for this condition?

Notes from Physical & History

Now click on **Physicians' Orders**.

 7. What orders are directly related to the treatment of KS? How does this compare with the typical medical intervention? In the left-hand column below, indicate the current orders, if any, for treatment of KS in Ira Bradley's chart. In the right-hand column, describe the typical treatment for KS affecting the integumentary system (see Table 14-2 in your textbook).

Orders for Ira Bradley	Treatment According to Textbook

 8. According to the textbook, there are three primary goals of cancer care. Circle the goal of care that is most appropriate for Ira Bradley at this point. Provide a rationale for your answer.

Cure   Control   Palliation

 9. The Red Rock Hospital Cancer Careplan lists the following nursing diagnoses. Indicate which are applicable to Ira Bradley's situation. For those not applicable as written, suggest modifications to make them specific to his needs.

Nursing Diagnosis	Applicable as Is? (Yes or No)	Suggested Modification
Impaired oral mucous membrane related to chemotherapy or radiation		

Nursing Diagnosis	Applicable as Is? (Yes or No)	Suggested Modification
Fatigue related to effects of cancer		
Ineffective coping related to depression secondary to diagnosis and treatment		
Disturbed body image related to hair loss, disfiguring surgery and weight loss		
Interupted family processes related to cancer diagnosis of family member		

LESSON 13

Fluid and Electrolyte Imbalance—Part I: Preclinical Preparation

Reading Assignment: Nursing Management: Fluid, Electrolyte, and Acid-Base Imbalances (Chapter 16)

Patient: Ira Bradley, Room 309

In this lesson, you will continue to care for Ira Bradley. Now you are interested in learning about his fluid and electrolyte status upon admission and the initial treatment for this.

CD-ROM Activity

Go to the Supervisor's Office and sign in to work with Ira Bradley for the Tuesday 0700 shift. Proceed to the Nurses' Station and open his chart. Read the entire Physical & History, including the Emergency Department Report.

Writing Activity

1. Below and on the next page, list data you found in the Emergency Department Report and other sections of the Physical & History that suggest a possible fluid and electrolyte imbalance. Are the findings consistent?

Emergency Department Report

Physical & History

2. The physician indicates Ira Bradley is dehydrated. What events most likely led to this condition?

➡ Now click on **Nurses' Notes** and read the note documented by T. Landers at 2335 Sunday.

3. What subjective and objective data are found, if any, that address Ira Bradley's fluid and electrolyte status?

Subjective Data

Objective Data

➤ Next, click on **Physicians' Orders** and read the orders for Sunday at 2255.

4. What lab tests were ordered that could provide important information regarding fluid and electrolyte status? In the presence of dehydration, what results are expected?

Lab tests useful for assessing fluid and electrolyte status	Expected results in presence of dehydration

5. In addition to the lab tests, what other orders written on Sunday night are specific interventions to manage dehydration?

➡ Close the chart and open Ira Bradley's EPR.

6. Find the lab results for the CBC, albumin, Chem 7, and urinalysis that were done on Sunday evening. Record the findings in the table below. Then indicate whether each value is low (L), high (H), or in the normal range (N). Finally, indicate what you think might be causing the change in value, if applicable.

Lab	Value	L, H, N	Meaning
Na$^+$			
K$^+$			
Cl$^-$			
CO$_2$			
BUN			
Creatinine			
Albumin			

Lab	Value	L, H, N	Meaning
Hgb			
Hct			
Urine specific gravity			

  7. Look at the figure below from your textbook. Based on the information you have collected so far, circle the box that best represents the pathology of Ira Bradley's fluid and electrolyte condition upon admission. Then circle the appropriate description of the cause of the problem.

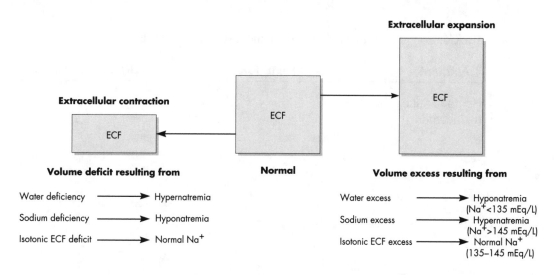

8. Ira Bradley has experienced a fluid shift. Fill in the sodium level in the space below. Next, draw an arrow indicating the direction of fluid shift between the extracellular space and the intracellular space.

Extracellular Fluid

Na⁺ level _____

Intracellular Fluid

Refer to your textbook regarding collaborative care in the treatment of hypernatremia to answer the following questions.

9. What is the primary goal of treatment?

10. Compare the treatment described in the textbook with Ira Bradley's orders.

Treatment	Textbook	Ira Bradley's Orders
Route of fluid replacement		
Type of IV fluid		

Now, consider intake and output (I&O).

11. What would you anticipate the I&O records to reflect over the first 24 to 48 hours of hospitalization? What would be a reasonable guess as to the intake verses the output? Would you expect these to be nearly equal?

12. What did the I&O actually look like? With the EPR still open, click on **I&O**. Record intake and output totals for the following time frames:

	Sunday Admission to 2400	Sunday 2400 to Monday 0800	Monday 0800 to 1600	Totals
Intake Totals				
Output Totals				

13. Are the totals similar to what you expected? How do the above totals compare with what you expected? How can you explain these totals?

→ Now click on **Assessment** (still in the EPR). Review the assessments completed by the nursing staff from admission until now (Tuesday 0700).

14. What data can be found that addresses the fluid and electrolyte status? From this standpoint, do you think the documentation is adequate? What could have been and/or should have been included as part of the nursing assessment?

→ Close the EPR. Go back to Ira Bradley's chart and review physicians' notes, physicians' orders, and nurses' notes from Sunday night until now, Tuesday morning.

15. What documentation and changes in orders, if any, reflect a change in the patient's care concerning his dehydration? Do any of the data seem surprising to you? If so, which? Record your answers below and on the next page.

Physicians' Notes   Monday:

Tuesday:

Physicians' Orders   Monday:

Tuesday:

Nurses' Notes Monday:

Tuesday:

Fluid and Electrolyte Imbalance—Part II

🔖 **Reading Assignment:** Nursing Management: Fluid, Electrolyte, and Acid-Base Imbalances (Chapter 16)

Patient: Ira Bradley, Room 309

In Lesson 13 you completed preclinical preparation for Ira Bradley, a 43-year-old man admitted to the hospital on Sunday with late-stage HIV infection, *Pneumocystis carinii* pneumonia, candidiasis, and Kaposi's sarcoma (KS). That lesson focused on the patient's fluid and electrolyte status upon admission and his initial treatment. In this lesson you will continue to follow this case as Ira Bradley recovers from dehydration.

💿 **CD-ROM Activity**

Go to the Supervisor's Office and sign in to work with Ira Bradley for the Tuesday 0700 shift. Proceed to the Nurses' Station and check the bulletin board to determine where report is being given for this patient. Go to that location and listen to the nursing report.

1. Below, record pertinent information from report regarding fluid and electrolyte status.

➡ Return to the Nurses' Station and open the MAR (in the blue notebook on the countertop).

2. What is the IV fluid and infusion rate being administered at this time?

3. What is the physiologic effect of this IV fluid?

4. If you have a 20 gtt/cc administration set, what is the correct drip rate (gtts/minute) to deliver the IV fluid at the ordered infusion rate?

5. If you know that a new liter of IV fluid was hung at 0400 this morning, about what time should you anticipate this liter will be empty?

→ Go to Ira Bradley's room to conduct the physical examination.

6. Record physical examination findings below. Include data that you think provide some information about fluid and electrolyte status. Also explain *how* each finding relates to fluid and electrolyte assessment.

Assessment findings related to fluid and electrolyte status	How do findings relate to fluid and electrolyte assessment?

7. What additional assessment would you perform to gain further information regarding the progress of Ira Bradley's hydration status or related treatment?

8. Your nursing instructor encourages you to consider using the nursing diagnosis Deficient Fluid Volume for your plan of care. Write this as a three-part nursing diagnosis.

Deficient fluid volume related to:

as manifested by:

9. One of the goals for Ira Bradley is rehydration. Interventions to accomplish this goal include administration of intravenous infusion of fluids and increased oral fluid intake. Considering these efforts, answer the following questions:

   a. What are some nursing interventions that can help increase the oral fluid intake, given the infection in his mouth?

   b. In what way does the management of Ira Bradley's fever, episodic diarrhea, and shortness of breath contribute to rehydration efforts?

   c. In what ways could you evaluate the effectiveness of the rehydration efforts?

It is now Friday and you have returned to the hospital to follow up on Ira Bradley. You are specifically interested in his fluid and electrolyte status and how his care may have changed since Tuesday. In the Supervisor's Office, sign in to work with him again, selecting Friday 0700 as your shift. Go to the Nurses' Station and open Ira Bradley's chart. Review the physicians' orders, physicians' notes, and nurses' notes for any indication regarding his condition, change in status, or change in orders that specifically address the fluid and electrolyte imbalance.

10. Record your findings below and on the next page.

Day	Data	Source (physicians' notes, physicians' orders, nurses' notes)
Tuesday		Physicians' notes
		Physicians' orders
		Nurses' notes
Wednesday		Physicians' notes
		Physicians' orders
		Nurses' notes

Day	Data	Source (physicians' notes, physicians' orders, nurses' notes)
Thursday		Physicians' notes
		Physicians' orders
		Nurses' notes

→ Close the patient's chart and move to the computer under the bookshelf. Access Ira Bradley's EPR and review his electrolytes and urine specific gravity over the entire week. (You will need to click on **Chemistry** and **Urinalysis** to find this data.)

11. Record your findings below and explain any changes in the data.

Test	Sunday	Tuesday	Thursday
Na^+			
K^+			
Cl^-			
CO_2			
BUN			
Creatinine			
Urine specific gravity			

Explanation for changes:

12. Now look at the intake and output totals over the entire week. Fill in the 24-hour I&O totals below. Explain any changes in the data.

Day	Intake totals	Output totals
Sunday		
Monday		
Tuesday		
Wednesday		
Thursday		

Explanation of changes:

→ Close Ira Bradley's EPR and return to his chart. Click on **Health Team**. As you read each health team member's report, consider the problems Ira Bradley was experiencing when he was admitted. To what extent is the reoccurrence of dehydration discussed?

13. Below and on the next page, indicate what each of the three health team members reported, if anything, regarding hydration.

Health Team Member	Information in Report Regarding Hydration
Sara Terney	

Health Team Member	Information in Report Regarding Hydration
Ray Burns	
Bridget Natalicio	

14. What strategies can you think of that would reduce Ira Bradley's chances of dehydration in the future?

LESSON 15 ──────────────────────────────

Perioperative Care

──────────────────────────────

Reading Assignment: Nursing Management: Preoperative Care (Chapter 17)
Nursing Management: Intraoperative Care (Chapter 18)
Nursing Management: Postoperative Care (Chapter 19)

Patient: David Ruskin, Room 303

In this lesson, you will be considering the perioperative experience of David Ruskin, who was struck by a motor vehicle while riding a bicycle, suffering a fractured right humerus and a closed head injury.

CD-ROM Activity

Go to the Supervisor's Office and sign in to work with David Ruskin for the Tuesday 0700 shift. Proceed to the Nurses' Station and open his chart. Read the Emergency Department Report in the Physical & History section.

1. What time did David Ruskin present to the Emergency Department?

2. What time did he go to surgery?

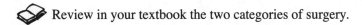 Review in your textbook the two categories of surgery.

3. Which type of surgery did David Ruskin have—elective or emergency? *(Circle one.)*

4. According to the textbook, three conditions must be met to obtain a valid consent for surgery.

   a. What are these three conditions?

b. Why did David Ruskin's wife Lisa sign the operative permit instead of David?

5. Your textbook describes several common fears associated with surgery. Which of the following, if any, are documented fears that David Ruskin had before going into surgery? (Place an **X** next to all that apply.)

_____ Fear of pain

_____ Fear of the unknown

_____ Fear of death

_____ Fear of anesthesia

_____ Fear of disruption of life patterns

 6. Read the section on assessment of the preoperative patient in your textbook. How does this compare with David Ruskin's preoperative assessment? Why are there differences?

7. If you had been the ER nurse caring for David Ruskin, what preoperative teaching would you have provided? How would his level of consciousness have affected your teaching?

8. Many patients receive preoperative medications, sometimes a single drug, sometimes a combination of drugs. Listed below and on the next page are common types of preoperative medications discussed in your textbook. Indicate the purpose for which these drugs are given.

Medication	Purpose
Benzodiazepines	
Anticholinergics	
Narcotics	

Medication	Purpose
Antiemetics	
Antibiotics	

→ Review the physicians' orders in David Ruskin's chart.

9. Which of the medications listed in question 8 were administered to this patient before his surgery?

→ Now review the surgeons' notes for David Ruskin.

10. According to the surgeons' notes, what time was he brought into the operating room?

11. What time did his surgery actually begin?

12. What surgical procedure was performed on David Ruskin?

13. How was the patient's fracture repaired?

14. What time did the surgical procedure end?

According to the report, David Ruskin was transferred to the Postanesthesia Care Unit (PACU) at 1855. Refer to your textbook to answer the following questions.

15. When a patient is admitted to the PACU, the major initial priority is assessment. What specific priorities are associated with this assessment?

16. In the PACU, nurses monitor for common respiratory complications such as airway obstruction, hypoxemia, and hypoventilation. What is the most common source of airway obstruction immediately after general anesthesia? What is the most common cause of hypoxemia?

17. What criteria must be met before a patient can be discharged from the PACU and transferred to the nursing unit?

→ David Ruskin was transferred from the PACU to the nursing unit at 2000. Immediately upon receiving this patient, the nurse performed an assessment. In David Ruskin's chart, read the nurses' notes for Sunday at 2030. Then close the chart and open David Ruskin's EPR. Click on **Assessment** and read the documentation regarding his initial postoperative assessment.

18. Compare the data you read in the nurses' notes and EPR with that shown in the table below from your textbook. What is your opinion of the assessment data documented by the nurses on the unit? Are their findings consistent with what is suggested in the table? Place a check mark next to each item below that is documented either in the EPR or the nurses' notes.

Nursing Assessment and Care of Patient on Admission to Clinical Unit
_____

- Record time of patient's return to unit
- Take baseline vital signs
    Assess airway and breath sounds
- Assess neurologic status, including level of consciousness and movement of extremities
- Assess wound, dressing, drainage tubes
    Note type and amount of drainage
    Connect tubing to gravity or suction drainage
- Assess color and appearance of skin
- Assess urinary status
    Note time of voiding
    Note presence of catheter and total output
    Check for bladder distention or urge to void
    Note catheter patency
- Assess pain and discomfort
    Note last dose and type of pain control
    Note current pain intensity
- Position for airway maintenance, comfort, safety (bed in low position, side rails up)
- Check IV infusion
    Note type of solution
    Note amount of fluid remaining
    Note flow rate
    Check integrity of insertion site and size of catheter
- Attach call light within reach and reorient patient to use of call light
- Ensure that emesis basin and tissues are available
- Determine emotional condition and support
    Check for presence of family member or significant other
- Check and carry out postoperative orders
_____

→ After completing an assessment, the nurse caring for David Ruskin should immediately review the physicians' orders and initiate a plan of care. Go back to the patient's chart, click on **Physicians' Orders** and read the Sunday 1930 postoperative orders. Next, review the Postoperative Care Plan in your textbook.

19. Based on the nursing postoperative assessment and physicians' orders, which of the following nursing diagnoses and collaborative problems seem applicable in David Ruskin's situation? (Circle all that apply.)

Nursing Diagnoses	Collaborative Problems
Pain	PC: Thromboembolism
Risk for infection	PC: Paralytic ileu
Anxiety	PC: Hemorrhage
Nausea	PC: Urinary retention
Ineffective airway clearance	
Risk for constipation	

20. What additional problems (nursing diagnoses or collaborative problems) would you include?

LESSON 16 ————————————————

Pneumonia—Part I: Preclinical Preparation

————————————————————————————

 Reading Assignment: Nursing Assessment: Respiratory System (Chapter 25)
Nursing Management: Lower Respiratory Problems
(Chapter 27)

Patient: Sally Begay, Room 304

In this lesson, you will complete preclinical preparation for Sally Begay, a 58-year-old Navajo woman with a diagnosis of pneumonia.

CD-ROM Activity

Go to the Supervisor's Office and sign in to work with Sally Begay for the Tuesday 0700 shift. Proceed to the Nurses' Station and open her chart. In the Physical & History, read the admitting report completed in the Emergency Department at 1200.

1. What was Sally Begay's initial admitting diagnosis?

2. Now scroll down to read the History of Present Illness section of the Physical & History. What are Sally Begay's primary symptoms, and how long has she had these symptoms?

157

3. What other health problems does Sally Begay have, according to her history? (*Hint: Five problems are listed under Significant Medical History.*)

→ An initial possible diagnosis for Sally Begay was Hantavirus. To answer the following questions, you will need to use sources other than your textbook. One good source is the CDC Website on Hantavirus. *(http://www.cdc.gov/ncidod/diseases/hanta/hps/).* You can access this site on the Intranet computer in the Nurses' Station.

4. What is Hantavirus?

5. What data are found in the History of Present Illness section that make the physician suspect the possibility of this diagnosis?

6. Sally Begay is ultimately diagnosed with pneumonia. Your textbook describes two classifications of pneumonia, based on how the infection was acquired. Which type of pneumonia does Sally Begay have?

7. Sally Begay is found to have bacterial pneumonia. Briefly describe the four stages of bacterial pneumonia, as described in your textbook.

Stage	Description
Congestion	
Red hepatization	
Gray hepatization	
Resolution	

8. On the flow sheet below, indicate where each of the four stages (congestion, red hepatization, gray hepatization, and resolution) occur. *(Note: Refer to Figure 27-1 in your textbook if you need help.)*

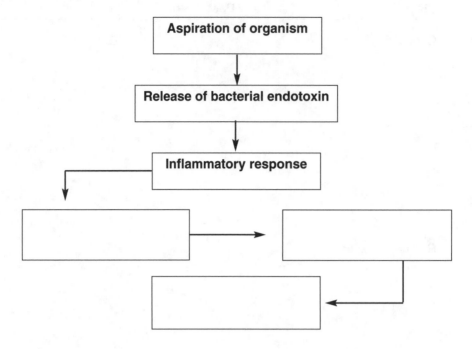

9. Which medical problem found in Sally Begay's medical history is most likely to have contributed to the development of pneumonia?
   a. MI 5 years ago
   b. Angina
   c. Hypertension
   d. Congestive heart failure
   e. COPD—chronic bronchitis

→ Click on **Physicians' Orders** in the patient's chart. Look over the initial orders written at 1230 on Saturday. Compare the diagnostic tests ordered with the common diagnostic measures for pneumonia presented in Table 27-5 in your textbook.

10. Which of the following diagnostic measures were ordered for Sally Begay? (Place an **X** next to all correct answers.)

   ____ History and physical examination   ____ Pulse oximetry or ABG

   ____ Chest x-ray   ____ CBC

   ____ Gram's stain of sputum   ____ Blood cultures

   ____ Sputum culture

→ Now click on **Diagnostics** in the chart. Read the CXR report by Dr. Kawasaki.

11. What findings appear on the x-ray that suggest pneumonia?

→ Close the chart and open Sally Begay's EPR (on the computer under the bookshelf).

12. Find the results of the CBC done on Saturday. In the chart below, write the normal value for each test. *(Note: Refer to Appendix B in your textbook for normal lab values.)* Then record Sally Begay's results for each test. Circle any abnormal values.

Test	Normal Value	Sally Begay's Results
Hgb		
Hct		
WBC		
RBC		
Platelets		

13. Now find the results of the ABG done on Saturday. Record Sally Begay's results below, as well as the normal value for each test. *(See Appendix B in your textbook.)* Circle any abnormal values.

Test	Normal Value	Sally Begay's Results
pH		
$PaCO_2$		
PaO_2		
HCO_3		

14. What is the significance of the CBC and ABG results? What do these results reflect?

→ Close the EPR and access Sally Begay's MAR (in the blue notebook on the counter).

15. Listed below are the medications (routine or PRN) ordered specifically to treat Sally Begay's pneumonia. Indicate the classification of each medication and the role you believe it plays in the treatment of pneumonia.

Medication	Type/Classification	Role in Treatment of Pneumonia
Erythromycin		
Ceftizoxime		
Acetaminophen		
Albuterol		

16. Why are two antibiotics ordered for Sally Begay? How do they differ? What are the specific indications for both of these antibiotics?

17. Make a list of the routine medications you will be administering during the day shift at each of the following times.

Time	Medications to Be Given
0900	
1200	
1400	

18. A change in the medication orders is documented on Sally Begay's MAR for today. Did you see this change in order? What change occurred? Where can you verify this change in order? Do you need to change the information you recorded in question 17?

19. The ceftizoxime is ordered to be given IVPB. Sally Begay has a primary intravenous infusion of D_5 1/2 NS. Is ceftizoxime compatible with this primary solution? How can you find out?

20. Since Sally Begay is capable of drinking fluids, why does she have an IV running at D_5 1/2 NS at 75 cc/hour?

LESSON 17

Pneumonia—Part II

/⌒⌒⌒ **Reading Assignment:** Nursing Assessment: Respiratory System (Chapter 25)
Nursing Management: Lower Respiratory System (Chapter 27)
Patient: Sally Begay, Room 304

In this lesson, you will continue working with Sally Begay, a 58-year-old Navajo woman with pneumonia. *(Note: You should have completed Lesson 16 prior to beginning this lesson.)*

CD-ROM Activity

Go to the Supervisor's Office and sign in to work with Sally Begay for the Tuesday 0700 shift. Proceed to the bulletin board in the Nurses' Station to determine where report is being given for this patient. Go to that location.

1. As you listen to the report on Sally Begay, complete the following report form.

Red Rock Canyon Medical Center
Report Notes

Patient: Room #

Age: Diagnosis:

Vital Signs:

O$_2$ Sat:

Pain:

Treatments:

Significant Assessment Findings:

IV Location/Date:

Identified Patient/Family Problems:

---

2. There were two errors in the report you heard. Compare your data in question 1 of this lesson with what you learned about Sally Begay in Lesson 16. What information given to you by the nurse is incorrect?

3. What is the significance of these errors in the report? Will they ultimately affect your nursing care? What should you do about these errors?

→ It is time to take the patient's vital signs. Go to Sally Begay's room and click on **Vital Signs**.

4. Collect a full set of measurements and record your findings below.

Heart rate:

Blood pressure:

Temperature:

Respiratory rate:

Oxygen saturation:

Pain:

5. What did you observe about the oxygen saturation procedure that could affect the accuracy of the measurement?

6. Consider the data you recorded in question 4. Which data are out of normal range? Is there any action you would consider taking? If so, explain.

→ It is now time to complete a physical examination. Click first on **Physical** and then on each of the three specific examination areas.

7. Record your data for each area of Sally Begay's physical examination below.

Physical Examination Area	Data
Head and Neck	
Chest/Upper Extremities	
Abdomen and Lower Extremities	

8. What findings collected from the physical examination are useful in evaluating Sally Begay's status in regards to the pneumonia? What additional data would you have also included, based on what you observed during the examination?

➤ It is now 1000, and you need to conduct a health history interview. Click first on the **Health History** icon. Then conduct your interview by selecting each of the 12 health pattern categories (one at a time) and clicking on the three question areas for each category.

9. Record *significant data* from Sally Begay's health history below and on the next pages.

Health History Area	Data
Perception/Self-Concept	

Activity

Health History Area	Data
Sexuality/Reproduction	
Culture	
Nutrition-Metabolic	
Sleep-Rest	

Health History Area	Data

Role/Relationship

Health Perception

Elimination

Cognitive/Perceptual

Health History Area	Data
Coping/Stress	
Value/Belief	

10. Compare Sally Begay's presenting symptoms and her physical findings with the nursing assessment data commonly associated with pneumonia, as presented in the table below (Table 27-6 from your textbook). Circle or highlight data that are similar to findings for Sally Begay.

Subjective Data
Important Health Information
  Past health history: Lung cancer, COPD, diabetes, chronic debilitating disease, malnutrition, altered consciousness, AIDS, exposure to chemical toxins, dust, or allergens
  Medications: Use of antibiotics; corticosteroids, chemotherapy, or any other immunosuppressants
  Surgeries or other treatment: Recent abdominal or thoracic surgery, splenectomy, endotracheal intubation, or any surgery with general anesthesia

Functional Health Patterns
  Health perception-health management: Cigarette smoking, alcoholism; recent upper respiratory tract infection, malaise
  Nutritional-metabolic: Anorexia, nausea, vomiting; chills
  Activity-exercise: Prolonged bed rest or immobility; fatigue, weakness; dyspnea, cough (productive or nonproductive); nasal congestion
  Cognitive-perceptual: Pain with breathing, chest pain, sore throat, headache, abdominal pain, muscle aches

Objective Data
General
  Fever, restlessness or lethargy; splinting of affected area

Respiratory
  Tachypnea; pharyngitis; asymmetric chest movements or retraction; decreased excursion; nasal flaring; use of accessory muscles (neck, abdomen); grunting; crackles, friction rub on auscultation; dullness on percussion over consolidated areas, increased tactile fremitus on palpation; pink, rusty, purulent, green, yellow, or white sputum (amount may be scant to copious)

Cardiovascular
  Tachycardia

Neurologic
  Changes in mental status, ranging from confusion to delirium

Possible Findings
  Leukocytosis; abnormal ABGs with decreased or normal PaO_2, decreased $PaCO_2$, and increased pH initially, and later decreased PaO_2, increased $PaCO_2$, and decreased pH; positive sputum Gram's stain and culture; patchy or diffuse infiltrates, abscesses, pleural effusion, or pneumothorax on chest x-ray

11. Based on the health history interview, physical examination findings, and data from the chart, develop a list of nursing diagnoses and a list of collaborative problems for Sally Begay. Be sure that everything on your lists can be supported with data. *(Note: Refer to the care plan in your textbook for additional help.)*

Nursing Diagnoses   **Collaborative Problems**

12. Review the lists you developed in question 11. Choose two nursing diagnoses or collaborative problems *not found* on the care plan in the textbook. Develop these further by identifying patient outcomes and nursing interventions specific to Sally Begay's situation. Why did you select the ones that you did?

Nursing Diagnosis or Collaborative Problem	Outcomes	Nursing Interventions

→ Your next task is to do some follow-up regarding Sally Begay's condition. To accomplish this we are going to take a "virtual leap in time" to Friday morning. Go back to the Supervisor's Office and sign in again. (Remember: You will have to click on **Reset** before you can switch shifts.) Keep Sally Begay as your patient, but change your duty time to Friday 1100. Although Sally Begay was discharged home earlier this morning, her chart remains. Go to the Nurses' Station and open her chart.

13. Open the physicians' notes and read the notes from Tuesday until discharge. What changes occurred during the rest of the week?

14. Now read the nurses' notes. What changes in Sally Begay's status are evident through the documentation in the nurses' notes?

 Review the pneumonia clinical pathway in your textbook.

COPD

👓 **Reading Assignment:** Nursing Assessment: Respiratory System (Chapter 25)
Nursing Management: Obstructive Pulmonary Diseases
(Chapter 28)
Patient: Sally Begay, Room 304

You have been assigned to care for Sally Begay, a 58-year-old Navajo woman with a diagnosis of pneumonia. This patient also has a long-standing history of bronchitis. If you have already completed Lessons 16 and 17, you may want to refer back to some of the data you collected as you complete this lesson.

💿 CD-ROM Activity

Go to the Supervisor's Office and sign in to work with Sally Begay for the Tuesday 0700 shift. Proceed to the Nurses' Station and open the patient's chart. In the Physical & History, read the admitting history completed in the Emergency Department at 1200. Next, close the chart and open Sally Begay's EPR. Read the entire Admissions Profile, which includes the nursing admission database.

1. How long has Sally Begay had bronchitis?

2. In addition to COPD and pneumonia, what other medical diagnoses does Sally Begay have?

3. Below, record the medications Sally Begay currently takes at home on a regular basis. Include the dosage and classification of each drug, as well as the reason the drug is taken.

Medication	Dose	Classification of Medication and Reason Taken

4. Based on her own medical history and her family history, what problem(s) is Sally Begay at risk for developing? Why?

In your textbook read the section on Emphysema and Chronic Bronchitis; then answer the following questions.

5. Define these terms: *chronic obstructive pulmonary disease*, *chronic bronchitis*, and *emphysema*.

Chronic obstructive pulmonary disease:

Chronic bronchitis:

Emphysema:

6. The textbook describes five major causes or etiologies of emphysema and chronic bronchitis. Below, identify those five etiologies, describe how each of these can lead to COPD, and indicate whether each etiology may have been a cause of chronic bronchitis for Sally Begay.

Etiology	Description of How This Can Lead to COPD

7. Based on the history in the patient's chart, which etiology or combination of etiologies seems most likely to have contributed to Sally Begay's COPD?

8. Briefly describe the pathophysiologic process of chronic bronchitis.

9. Draw a flow diagram of the pathophysiology of bronchitis.

10. What is the relationship between Sally Begay's primary admitting diagnosis (pneumonia) and the underlying chronic condition (chronic bronchitis)?

➤ Return to Sally Begay's chart, click on **Diagnostics**, and read the radiologic report by Dr. Kawasaka.

11. What findings on the CXR are consistent with COPD?

➤ Now flip back to the Physical & History. (Use the **Flip Back** icon in the lower right side of screen).

12. What was Sally Begay's arterial oxygen saturation in the Emergency Department? What is the normal range for oxygen saturation?

Sally Begay's O$_2$ Sat   **Normal Range O$_2$ Sat**

13. What exactly does an arterial oxygen saturation reflect? Why do you think her oxygen saturation deviates from normal?

→ Click on **Physicians' Orders**. Review the initial orders for Sally Begay written on Sunday
night.

14. The physician ordered oxygen therapy. What was the order? What percentage of oxygen
does this deliver?

15. What is the rationale for this oxygen order as opposed to high-flow oxygen administration
to relieve the hypoxia?

16. Which of the medications listed is specific for treatment of COPD? What is the action of
this drug? Describe how it is administered.

→ Now click on **Nurses' Notes** and read the notes for Saturday.

17. What problems have been identified by the nurse? What interventions have been planned? How do you think the effectiveness of these interventions will be evaluated? Record your answers below.

Identified Problems	Planned Interventions	How will these be evaluated?

18. Compare the identified problems and the planned interventions in the nurses' notes with the Nursing Care Plan in your textbook. What additional problems do you think should be included, based on what you know about Sally Begay?

→ Close Sally Begay's chart. Go to the computer under the bookshelf and access the EPR. Open Sally Begay's EPR and click on **Assessment**.

19. Compare the nursing assessment findings for Saturday at 1600 with those on Tuesday at 0400. Record your findings below.

Assessment Areas	Saturday 1600	Tuesday 0400
Temperature		
Heart rate		
Respiration		
Oxygen saturation		
Use of oxygen		
Respiratory pattern		
Lung fields		
Cough		
Sputum		

20. Based on the above assessment findings, how successful do you think the nursing interventions have been up to this point? What additional information would you want to consider?

21. What further interventions might be helpful in Sally Begay's case?

→ Now we are going to move forward in time to Thursday. Return to the Supervisor's Office to sign in again. Keep Sally Begay as your patient, but change your duty time to Thursday 1100.

22. By Thursday afternoon Sally Begay is getting ready for discharge. Go to the Nurses' Station and find the location of the health team meeting. Attend the meeting and take notes as you listen.

Reporting	Important Data
Rose Simpson, RN Nurse Case Manager	
Louise Johnson, RN Clinical Nurse Specialist	
Kris Holmes, MSW Social Worker	

23. Consider the health team report you just heard. Now compare your notes with the Ambulatory and Home Care section in the textbook. Review Table 28-24 (Patient and Family Teaching Guide) as well. Were the discharge concerns for Sally Begay consistent with the textbook information? Is there anything else you would want to include in your discharge planning for this patient?

Coronary Artery Disease

📖 **Reading Assignment:** Nursing Assessment: Cardiovascular System (Chapter 31)
Nursing Management: Coronary Artery Disease and Acute
Coronary Syndrome (Chapter 33)

Patient: Sally Begay, Room 304

Sally Begay is a 58-year-old Navajo woman with a diagnosis of pneumonia and chronic bronchitis. She also has a history of hypertension and coronary artery disease, a myocardial infarction 5 years ago, and mild CHF. You have been assigned to review this patient's chart to learn more about coronary artery disease.

💿 **CD-ROM Activity**

Go to the Supervisor's Office and sign in to work with Sally Begay for the Thursday 1100 shift. Proceed to the Nurses' Station and open her chart. In the Physical & History, read the admitting history completed in the Emergency Department at 1200.

1. Consider the risk factors for CAD. Identify each of the following risk factors as either unmodifiable (mark with a **U**) or modifiable (mark with an **M**). Circle those risk factors that are present in Sally Begay's history.

_____ Age   _____ Family history

_____ Elevated serum lipids   _____ Smoking

_____ Inactivity   _____ Hypertension

_____ Obesity   _____ Race

_____ Gender   _____ Stress/behavior patterns

 In your textbook, read the Clinical Manifestations of Coronary Artery Disease section. The textbook describes three clinical manifestations of CAD: angina, acute coronary syndrome, and sudden cardiac death.

2. Sally Begay has intermittent angina. What is angina?

3. Describe what happens during an angina episode.

4. List at least five different factors that could precipitate myocardial ischemia and angina pain.

5. According to Sally Begay's history, how often does she have angina chest pain?

6. What medication does Sally Begay have at home in case she has angina? How does this drug work to treat angina?

7. Which of the three types of angina does Sally Begay most likely have? (Circle one.)

      Stable angina   Unstable angina   Prinzmetal's angina

8. Sally Begay had a myocardial infarction (MI) 5 years ago. What is a myocardial infarction? Describe what happens during a myocardial infarction.

9. What is the relationship between having HTN and developing an MI?

10. What is the relationship between having an MI and developing CHF?

11. Read the Women and Coronary Artery Disease section in your textbook (near the end of Chapter 33). Describe how this information is consistent with Sally Begay's history.

→ Click on **Physicians' Orders** in Sally Begay's chart. The physician has ordered ECG monitoring.

12. What does this mean? Why has this been ordered?

13. Based on this order, what should the nurses include in their documentation?

→ Now open the nurses' notes and read the notes for Saturday through Wednesday evening.

14. What do the nurses' notes reflect regarding the cardiac monitoring?

15. Nearly all of the nurses' notes indicate that Sally Begay says she has pain in her chest. How can the nurse differentiate chest pain from angina, chest pain from a myocardial infarction, and chest pain from pneumonia?

→ You are asked by your nursing instructor to prepare patient teaching for Sally Begay. You decide to teach her about a healthy-heart diet as nutrition therapy education for coronary artery disease. First you need to collect pertinent data. Go into Sally Begay's room and click on **Health History**. Gather data in functional health pattern categories that you think will be helpful in your planning.

16. List pertinent data you collected from Sally Begay's health history interview that will help you plan your patient teaching.

17. What additional questions would you like to ask Sally Begay? What additional information would be helpful?

 18. Refer to Table 33-4 (Coronary Artery Disease Nutritional Therapy) in your textbook. How does this diet compare with what you know about Sally Begay's reported diet?

19. Would Table 33-4 be appropriate to use as a guide to teach Sally Begay about CAD nutrition? Discuss some of the pros and cons of using this table.

21

Congestive Heart Failure— Part I: Tuesday

/∞∅ **Reading Assignment:** Nursing Management: Heart Failure and Cardiomyopathy
(Chapter 34)
Patient: Carmen Gonzales, Room 302

For this lesson, you have been assigned to care for Carmen Gonzales, a 56-year-old female admitted to the hospital with a severe leg infection. She also has a history of type 2 diabetes mellitus, coronary artery disease (CAD), congestive heart failure (CHF), and hypertension.

Before you begin, review the pathophysiologic factors associated with CHF.

1. CHF typically manifests as:
   a. right-sided failure.
   b. left-sided failure.
   c. biventricular failure.

2. The most common form of initial heart failure is:
   a. right-sided failure.
   b. left-sided failure.
   c. biventricular failure.

3. Compare and contrast the most common causes of chronic and acute CHF below.

Chronic   **Acute**

4. On the figure below, complete the following activities:

a. Illustrate normal blood flow through the heart. Draw arrows to represent flow.
b. Illustrate afterload. Write the word *afterload* (to represent hypertension) next to the descending aorta.
c. Illustrate the backup of fluid from the left side of the heart (left ventricle) into the pulmonary vein and into the lungs.
d. Illustrate pulmonary edema by drawing dots or small circles on the lungs to show the location of excess fluid.
e. Illustrate the backup of fluid from the pulmonary artery into the right side of the heart and then into the peripheral system (superior and inferior vena cava).

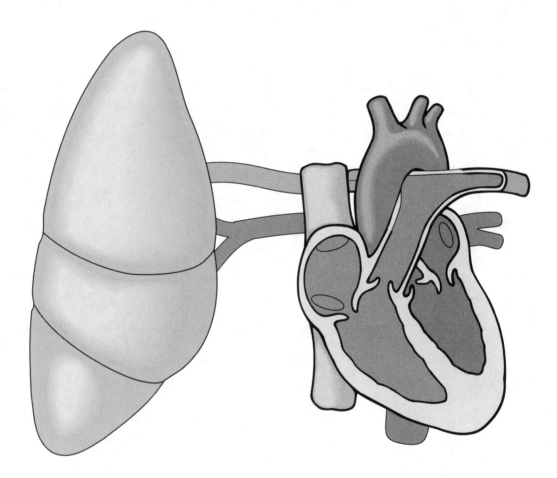

💿 CD-ROM Activity

Go to the Supervisor's Office and sign in to work with Carmen Gonzales for the Tuesday 0700 shift. Go to the Nurses' Station and open her chart. Read the Physical & History, including the Emergency Department Record. (Remember to scroll down to read all pages.)

5. What information is found in the Physical & History that specifically addresses Carmen Gonzales and her CHF?

6. If you had done the initial ER assessment of Carmen Gonzales, what additional history or examination would you have included specifically to assess the status of her CHF?

7. Your textbook identifies several risk factors for the development of CHF. Compare this information with the data found in Carmen Gonzales' chart. Below and on the next page, indicate whether Carmen Gonzales has each of the listed risk factors. Then record the data from the patient's chart that support your opinion.

Risk Factors	Does Carmen Gonzales have this risk factor?	What data support your answer?
Advancing age		
Coronary artery disease		
Hypertension		
Diabetes		

Risk Factors	Does Carmen Gonzales have this risk factor?	What data support your answer?
Smoking		
Obesity		
Elevated cholesterol levels		

→ Close Carmen Gonzales' chart. Access her EPR and read the Admissions Profile.

8. What data in the profile provide clues regarding the presence of symptoms of CHF?

→ Close the EPR and return to the patient's chart. Click on **Physicians' Orders** and review the orders for Carmen Gonzales.

9. What orders are present in Carmen Gonzales' chart that specifically address monitoring and management of her congestive heart failure?

→ The night nurse is ready to start report on Carmen Gonzales. Close the patient's chart and go to hear the report. (Remember: You can find out where report is being given by checking the bulletin board or by moving your cursor across the animated map.)

10. What did you think about the report you were given? Is there anything you wished the nurse would have included in the report regarding Carmen Gonzales' CHF? If so, what? The nurse in the report suggested you keep a close eye on the patient. How will you do this? What will you watch for? (Refer to Table 34-3 in your textbook for help.)

→ It is now 0745. Go inside Carmen Gonzales' room and click on **Vital Signs**.

11. Obtain a set of vital signs and record your findings below.

Temperature _____   Respiration _____

Heart rate _____   Blood pressure _____

Pain rating _____   Oxygen saturation _____

12. Consider the vital signs you just obtained. Are there any that concern you? If so, which one(s)?

→ Go to the Nurses' Station and access the EPR for Carmen Gonzales. Click on **Vital Signs**.

13. Review the vital sign data for Carmen Gonzales for the last couple of days and compare it with your findings in question 11. What would be the appropriate action by the nurse in this situation?

Return to Carmen Gonzales' room. Conduct a health history and physical examination, focusing particularly on data suggesting CHF.

14. The table below lists common assessment findings for CHF.

   a. Circle any data that you know from her history or that you collected during your assessment of Carmen Gonzales.

Table 21-1   Congestive Heart Failure

Subjective Data	Objective Data
Important Health Information	**Integumentary**
Past health history: CAD (including recent MI), hypertension, cardiomyopathy, valvular or congenital heart disease, diabetes mellitus, thyroid or lung disease, rapid or irregular heartbeat	Cool, diaphoretic skin; cyanosis or pallor, peripheral edema (right-sided heart failure)
Medications: Use of and compliance with any cardiac medications; use of diuretics, estrogens, corticosteroids, phenylbutazone, nonsteroidal antiinflammatory drugs	**Respiratory** Tachypnea, crackles, rhonchi, wheezes; frothy, blood-tinged sputum
	Cardiovascular Tachycardia, S_3, S_4, murmurs; pulsus alternans, PMI displaced inferiorly and posteriorly, jugular vein distention
Functional Health Patterns *Health perception-health management:* Fatigue *Nutritional-metabolic:* Usual sodium intake; nausea, vomiting, anorexia, stomach bloating; weight gain	**Gastrointestinal** Abdominal distention, hepatosplenomegaly, ascites
Elimination: Nocturia, decreased daytime urinary output, constipation *Activity-exercise:* Dyspnea, orthopnea, cough; palpitations; dizziness, fainting *Sleep-rest:* Number of pillows used for sleeping; paroxysmal nocturnal dyspnea	**Neurologic** Restlessness, confusion, decreased attention or memory
Cognitive-perceptual: Chest pain or heaviness; RUQ pain, abdominal discomfort; behavioral changes	**Possible Findings** Altered serum electrolytes (especially Na^+ and K^+), elevated BUN, creatinine, or liver function tests; chest x-ray demonstrating cardiomegaly, pulmonary congestion, and interstitial pulmonary edema; echocardiogram showing increased chamber size and decreased wall motion; atrial and ventricular enlargement on ECG; ↑ PAP, ↑ PAWP, ↓ CO, ↓ CI, ↓ O_2 saturation, ↑ SVR on hemodynamic monitoring

15. Based on what you have assessed, identify from the following list the most significant priorities for Carmen Gonzales for the rest of your shift. (Place an **X** next to all diagnoses or collaborative problems that apply at this time.)

_____ Pain   _____ Risk for impaired gas exchange

_____ Risk for fall   _____ Ineffective therapeutic regimen management

_____ Activity intolerance   _____ Impaired skin integrity

_____ Deficient fluid volume   _____ Risk for ineffective role performance

_____ PC: Pulmonary edema   _____ PC: Increased intracranial pressure

22

Congestive Heart Failure— Part II: Thursday

Reading Assignment: Nursing Management: Heart Failure and Cardiomyopathy
(Chapter 34)

Patient: Carmen Gonzales, Room 302

For this lesson, you will continue your assignment for Carmen Gonzales, a 56-year-old female admitted to the hospital with a severe leg infection. She also has a history of type 2 DM, coronary artery disease (CAD), congestive heart failure (CHF), and hypertension. You should complete Lesson 21 prior to beginning this lesson.

CD-ROM Activity

Go to the Supervisor's Office and sign in to work with Carmen Gonzales for the Thursday 0700 shift. Before you visit your patient, go to the Nurses' Station and review her chart to determine changes in her status since you cared for her on Tuesday. Click on **Nurses' Notes** and read the notes for Tuesday afternoon and Wednesday.

1. Now that you have read the nurses' notes in Carmen Gonzales' chart, list below any significant data you found regarding CHF.

2. Now read the physicians' orders. Record the orders for Tuesday afternoon below.

→ Next, click on **Diagnostics** in Carmen Gonzales' chart.

3. Read and record the radiology report for Tuesday afternoon.

4. Read the cardiology consultation for Tuesday and Wednesday. What do these findings show?

5. According to her chart, Carmen Gonzales had a short episode of right-sided CHF caused by fluid volume overload after you left the hospital on Tuesday afternoon. What specific signs and symptoms did she have that are consistent with a diagnosis of right-sided heart failure? On the table below, put an asterisk (*) next to any data you collected from the cardiology report, radiology report, or nurses' notes in the patient's chart.

Subjective Data

Important Health Information

Past health history: CAD (including recent MI), hypertension, cardiomyopathy, valvular or congenital heart disease, diabetes mellitus, thyroid or lung disease, rapid or irregular heartbeat
Medications: Use of and compliance with any cardiac medications; use of diuretics, estrogens, corticosteroids, phenylbutazone, nonsteroidal antiinflammatory drugs

Functional Health Patterns

Health perception-health management: Fatigue
Nutritional-metabolic: Usual sodium intake; nausea, vomiting, anorexia, stomach bloating; weight gain
Elimination: Nocturia, decreased daytime urinary output, constipation
Activity-exercise: Dyspnea, orthopnea, cough; palpitations; dizziness, fainting
Sleep-rest: Number of pillows used for sleeping; paroxysmal nocturnal dyspnea
Cognitive-perceptual: Chest pain or heaviness; RUQ pain, abdominal discomfort; behavioral changes

Objective Data

Integumentary

Cool, diaphoretic skin; cyanosis or pallor, peripheral edema (right-sided heart failure)

Respiratory

Tachypnea, crackles, rhonchi, wheezes; frothy, blood-tinged sputum

Cardiovascular

Tachycardia, S_3, S_4, murmurs; pulsus alternans, PMI displaced inferiorly and posteriorly, jugular vein distention

Gastrointestinal

Abdominal distention, hepatosplenomegaly, ascites

Neurologic

Restlessness, confusion, decreased attention or memory

Possible Findings

Altered serum electrolytes (especially Na^+ and K^+), elevated BUN, creatinine, or liver function tests; chest x-ray demonstrating cardiomegaly, pulmonary congestion, and interstitial pulmonary edema; echocardiogram showing increased chamber size and decreased wall motion; atrial and ventricular enlargement on ECG; ↑ PAP, ↑ PAWP, ↓ CO, ↓ CI, ↓ O_2 saturation, ↑ SVR on hemodynamic monitoring

→ Close the chart and access the EPR for Carmen Gonzales. Click on **I&O**.

6. Review the intake and output records since Carmen Gonzales' admission. Calculate the following information:

	Total Intake	Total Output
Sunday		
Monday		
Tuesday through 1500		
3-day totals		

7. What conclusions can be made regarding the findings recorded in question 6?

8. Explain the signs and symptoms Carmen Gonzales has experienced from a pathophysiologic perspective. How did fluid volume overload cause her symptoms?

As you know, the physician ordered furosemide 20 mg IV stat on Tuesday afternoon. Use a nursing drug reference to answer the following questions.

9. What is the action of furosemide? (In other words, how does it work, and on what part of the kidney does its action take place?)

10. What is the desired therapeutic effect of furosemide? How could the nurse assess whether this desired effect was achieved?

11. Why would furosemide be the diuretic of choice to use in this situation, as opposed to a thiazide diuretic? Why was it given IV instead of orally?

12. Refer again to the intake and output record in the EPR. What happened to the urine output after the furosemide was administered? Now calculate the 24-hour I&O totals for Sunday through Wednesday.

	Total Intake	Total Output
Sunday		
Monday		
Tuesday		
Wednesday		
3-day totals		

13. What conclusions can be made regarding the data you recorded in question 12?

→ Close the EPR notes and open Carmen Gonzales' MAR (in the blue notebook on the counter).

14. Determine what routine medications you will be giving to Carmen Gonzales today during your shift (0700 to 1500). Below, list the medication(s) you need to give and the time each is due.

Medication	Why Given	Time Due

15. Now find out where the night nurse is giving report on Carmen Gonzales. Go to that location and listen to report. Record any pertinent information below.

16. Did you notice any discrepancies in the report from what you read in the chart? If so, explain.

→ It is now 0745. Go to Carmen Gonzales' room and click on **Vital Signs**.

17. Obtain a set of vital signs and record your findings below.

Temperature _____   Respiration _____

Heart rate _____   Blood pressure _____

Pain rating _____   Oxygen saturation _____

→ Go to the Nurses' Station and open the EPR for Carmen Gonzales. Record the vital signs. Close the EPR.

It is 0800. Return to Carmen Gonzales' room. Click on **Medications** and administer the 0800 medications to the patient.

Your nursing instructor suggests that you participate in Carmen Gonzales' discharge planning and patient teaching. To prepare for this, do the following:

- Go to the discharge planning meeting today (see the bulletin board in the Nurses' Station for location.)
- Review the Physical & History and the health team reports in the patient's chart.
- Consider the data you collected during your interview and examination on Tuesday (review these again if needed).
- Review the data in the Admissions Profile in Carmen Gonzales' EPR.

18. What specific issues have you identified from Carmen Gonzales' data that may influence how you approach her discharge teaching?

19. How does Carmen Gonzales' ethnicity factor into her discharge teaching?

→ Your instructor suggests that you briefly teach Carmen Gonzales about low-sodium diets. (The dietitian will spend time with her prior to discharge specifically to develop a menu plan with her that addresses DM and CHF.) You decide to go over four points about low-sodium diets.

20. Using Tables 34-9, 34-10, and 34-11 from your textbook, complete the following teaching instruction sheet for Carmen Gonzales.

- What is a low-sodium diet?

- Why is a low-sodium diet important for you to follow?

- Many of the foods that you currently enjoy can be included on this diet. They are:

- There are several foods that should be avoided, if possible, on this diet. Examples include:

After teaching Carmen Gonzales about the low-sodium diet, your instructor suggests that you review the CHF Patient and Family Teaching Guide with her (Table 34-13 in your textbook).

21. In what way would you tailor the CHF teaching guide to meet Carmen Gonzales' needs?

Part VI—Problems of Ingestion, Digestion, Absorption, and Elimination

LESSON 23

Nutritional Problems

Reading Assignment: Nursing Management: Nutritional Problems (Chapter 39)
Patient: Ira Bradley, Room 309

For this lesson, you will apply nutrition concepts to the case of Ira Bradley. Ira is a 43-year-old male admitted to the hospital with a diagnosis of late-state HIV infection, *Pneumocystis carinii* pneumonia, candidiasis, and Kaposi's sarcoma.

CD-ROM Activity

Go to the Supervisor's Office and sign in to work with Ira Bradley for the Thursday 0700 shift. Proceed to the Nurses' Station and open his chart. Read the Emergency Department Report in the Physical & History.

1. What problems related to nutrition are evident by reading the Emergency Department Report?

2. Why do conditions such as HIV infection contribute to weight loss?

225

Copyright © 2004 by Mosby, Inc. All rights reserved.

Several anthropometric measurements are useful in evaluating nutritional status.

3. Look again at the Emergency Department Report for Ira Bradley. What are his admission height and weight?

Height _____

Weight _____

4. What is body mass index (BMI)? What is the normal or ideal, BMI range?

5. Determine Ira Bradley's BMI using the nomogram in your textbook (Figure 39-7).

BMI = _____

6. What does Ira Bradley's BMI reflect?

Biochemical or laboratory tests are also helpful in evaluation of nutritional status. In Ira Bradley's chart, review the initial physicians' orders written on Sunday night.

7. What laboratory test was done that is helpful to understand the patient's current status?

8. Compare Ira Bradley's admission albumin level with the normal range as given in Table 39-10 in your textbook.

Ira Bradley's level _____

Normal range _____

9. What does Ira Bradley's lab value indicate?

10. What is the difference between albumin and prealbumin levels?

 It should be obvious to you by now that Ira Bradley suffers from malnutrition. Refer to the textbook and read about nutritional needs of patients with physical illness.

11. According to your textbook, how does fever affect metabolic rate and nutritional needs?

→ 12. Close the patient's chart and open the EPR. Click on **Vital Signs**; then record Ira Bradley's temperature for the first 24 hours after admission.

Sunday 2400 _____   Monday 1200 _____

Monday 0400 _____   Monday 1600 _____

Monday 0800 _____   Monday 2000 _____

13. How much of an increase in BMR would you estimate Ira Bradley experienced the first 24 hours?

Clearly, a goal of nursing care for Ira Bradley's is to improve his nutritional status. Let's evaluate his nutritional intake during this hospitalization.

→ 14. How many calories do you think Ira Bradley took in between admission and Tuesday morning (before breakfast)? You won't find this specific information on the chart, but you can make an educated guess by completing the following steps:

a. An IV fluid was ordered for Ira Bradley upon admission. What specifically was the order? (If you don't remember, go back to his chart and review the physicians' orders.)

b. How many calories are in 1 liter of the IV fluid he received? (You may have to look in other sources for this information.)

c. Go back to the EPR and click on **I&0**. Approximately how much IV fluid did Ira Bradley receive during the first 24 hours since admission (Sunday 2400 to Monday 2400)?

d. Approximately how many total calories did Ira Bradley receive from the IV fluid? Record this in the chart below.

e. What meal(s) did Ira Bradley eat during the first 24 hours since admission? What percentage of his meal(s) did he intake during that time? (In the EPR, click on **ADL**, then on **Appetite**.) What is your best guess of total calories he consumed in the meal(s)? Record this in the chart below.

f. What would you estimate as Ira Bradley's total caloric intake between Sunday 2400 and Tuesday 0800? Record this below.

g. The clinical dietician tells you that for a 150-lb man with an infection, the caloric needs are over 4500 Kcal/day. Calculate the net difference between Ira Bradley's caloric needs and his actual intake during this time. Record this below.

Total calories from IV   _____

Estimated calories from   _____
meals (not including
Tuesday's breakfast)

Estimated caloric intake   _____
(Sunday 2400–
Tuesday 0800)

Estimated caloric needs   _____
per 24 hours

Net difference between   _____
caloric needs and
actual intake

15. What is your assessment of Ira Bradley's intake as recorded in question 14?

16. Review Ira Bradley's eating patterns for the rest of the week. What pattern of intake do you see, based on documentation in the EPR?

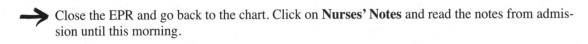

Close the EPR and go back to the chart. Click on **Nurses' Notes** and read the notes from admission until this morning.

17. Do the nurses' notes address Ira Bradley's nutritional status adequately? Explain.

 18. Review the various types of supplemental nutrition (tube feedings and parenteral nutrition) described in your textbook. Should any of these measures have been implemented?

19. What suggestions might you make to Ira Bradley and his wife regarding improvement of his nutritional status once he goes home?

LESSON **24**

Diabetes Mellitus—
Part I: Tuesday

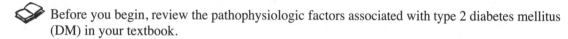 **Reading Assignment:** Nursing Assessment: Endocrine System (Chapter 46)

Nursing Management: Diabetes Mellitus (Chapter 47)

Patient: Carmen Gonzales, Room 302

For this lesson, you are assigned to care for Carmen Gonzales, a 56-year-old female patient admitted to the hospital with type 2 diabetes mellitus and a leg infection.

Before you begin, review the pathophysiologic factors associated with type 2 diabetes mellitus (DM) in your textbook.

1. What three metabolic abnormalities have a role in the development of type 2 diabetes?

2. Complete the following chart, comparing and contrasting the characteristics of type 1 and type 2 diabetes mellitus.

Characteristics	Type 1 Diabetes Mellitus	Type 2 Diabetes Mellitus
Age of onset		
Causes		
Symptoms at onset		
Use of insulin		
Use of oral hypoglycemic agents		
Common complications		

CD-ROM Activity

Go to the Supervisor's Office and sign in to work with Carmen Gonzales for the Tuesday 0700 shift. Before you visit the patient, go to the Nurses' Station and briefly review parts of her chart. Read the entire History & Physical, including the Emergency Department Record (Remember to scroll down to read all pages.)

3. What data in the chart specifically address Carmen Gonzales and her diabetes?

4. If you had done the initial ER assessment of Carmen Gonzales, what additional history or examination would you have included?

5. According to her medical history, Carmen Gonzales has coronary artery disease, hypertension, and congestive heart failure, and she had a severe right leg infection within the last 5 months. Is there a relationship between her diabetes and these other problems? If so, what might they be? Record your answers below and on the next page.

Medical Diagnosis	Relationship to Type 2 Diabetes Mellitus
Coronary artery disease	
Hypertension	

Medical Diagnosis	Relationship to Type 2 Diabetes Mellitus
Congestive heart failure	
Infection to leg	

 6. The textbook describes the clinical picture of type 2 diabetes mellitus. Fill in the following chart, comparing data from the textbook with data found in the Carmen Gonzales' Physical & History. Does she fit the clinical picture?

Clinical Picture	Textbook Description	Carmen Gonzales' Data	Fits Description? (Yes or No)
Age of onset			
Ethnicity			
Obesity			
Familial factors			

→ Click on **Physicians' Orders** and review the orders for Carmen Gonzales.

7. What orders are present that specifically address management of her diabetes?

→ Now click on **Expired MARs** and review this data.

8. How many times has insulin been given to Carmen Gonzales? At what dose(s)?

9. Carmen Gonzales does not take insulin at home. Why has it been ordered for this hospitalization? Why does she suddenly need it now?

10. As part of your clinical preparation, research information about glyburide in your textbook or your drug reference. Complete the following drug card based on your research.

DRUG CARD

Generic Name: Glyburide

Common Trade Names:

Mechanism of Action:

Dosage:

Administration Routes:

→ Close the patient's chart and access Carmen Gonzales' current MAR (in the blue notebook on the counter).

11. Determine what routine medications you will be administering to Carmen Gonzales today during the day shift (0700–1500). Below, list the routine medication(s) you need to give her, the reason why the med(s) will be given, and the time the med(s) should be given.

Medication	Why Given	Time Due

→ The nurse from the previous shift is ready to give report on Carmen Gonzales. Close the MAR, find out where report is being given, and go to hear report.

12. What did you think about the report you were given? Is there anything you wished the nurse would have included in the report regarding the patient's DM? If so, what?

→ It is now 0745. Go inside Carmen Gonzales' room and click on **Vital Signs**. Obtain a set of vital signs, and record your findings in the EPR. (You will need to leave the patient's room and go to one of the computers that access the EPR.)

13. Based on what you learned from obtaining vital signs, you should return to Carmen Gonzales' room and administer a PRN medication. What medication is appropriate? Why?

→ It is now time to give Carmen Gonzales her 0800 medications. Return to her room and click on **Medications** to complete this activity.

14. Consider administration guidelines associated with administration of glyburide. What is the rationale for administering glyburide at 0800? (You may need to refer to your nursing drug book.)

15. You learn from the charge nurse that Carmen Gonzales was given 6 units of regular SQ at 0730 (while you were listening to report) for a blood sugar of 260. Refer to your drug book or the textbook, and fill in the following information regarding regular insulin.

	Expected Length of Time	**Actual Time After 0730 Dose**
Onset		
Peak		
Duration		

→ You are now ready to conduct a physical examination of Carmen Gonzales. Click on **Physical** and obtain data in the three assessment areas.

16. Record your physical examination findings below and on the next page. Then go to the EPR and record the findings there as well.

Assessment	**Finding**
Head and Neck	
Chest/Upper Extremities	

Assessment	Finding
Abdomen and Lower Extremities	

17. Do any of your findings deviate from what you expected?

LESSON 25

Diabetes Mellitus—
Part II: Thursday

📖 **Reading Assignment:** Nursing Management: Diabetes Mellitus (Chapter 47)
Patient: Carmen Gonzales, Room 302

For this lesson, you will continue to care for Carmen Gonzales, a 56-year-old female patient admitted to the hospital with type 2 diabetes mellitus and a leg infection. You should complete Lesson 24 before beginning this lesson.

💿 **CD-ROM Activity**

Go to the Supervisor's Office and sign in to work with Carmen Gonzales for the Thursday 0700 shift. Proceed to the Nurses' Station and open the patient's chart. Briefly review parts of the chart to update you regarding her care since Tuesday. Specifically, review the expired MARs, physicians' notes, physicians' orders, and nurses' notes. When you are finished, close the chart and access Carmen Gonzales' MAR. Determine what routine medications you will be giving to Carmen Gonzales today during the day shift (0700–1500).

1. Below, list the routine medication(s) you need to give this patient. Also explain why you need to give the med(s) and record the time you need to administer the med(s).

Medication	Why Given	Time Due

2. When and why did the physician order furosemide for Carmen Gonzales? What effect could it have related to her diabetes? (Refer to a nursing drug book or your textbook for help.)

The night nurse is ready to give report on Carmen Gonzales. Close the MAR and check the bulletin board for the location of the report. Go there and listen to report.

3. What did you think about the report you were given? Is there anything you wished the nurse would have included in the report regarding Carmen Gonzales' DM? If so, what?

4. It is almost 0800. Go into Carmen Gonzales' room and obtain a set of vital signs. Record your findings below and in the EPR.

Heart rate _____

Respiration _____

Blood pressure _____

Temperature _____

Oxygen saturation _____

Pain rating _____

Return to Carmen Gonzales' room and administer her 0800 medications.

Your nursing instructor has asked that you participate in Carmen Gonzales' discharge planning. Before you do this, you need to collect more data. In the patient's room, click on **Health History** and conduct a patient interview. Specifically, pay attention to information that would be helpful in developing a plan of care for her at discharge, focusing on the diabetes.

5. Below and on the next two pages, record the data you have collected from the health history interview that will help you as you develop a plan of care for Carmen Gonzales.

Health History Area	Data
Perception/Self-Concept	
Activity	
Sexuality/Reproductive	
Culture	
Nutrition-Metabolic	

Health History Area	Data
Sleep-Rest	
Role/Relationship	
Health Perception	
Elimination	
Cognitive/Perceptual	
Coping/Stress	

Health History Area	Data

Value/Belief

6. What specific issues have you identified from Carmen Gonzales' medical history, interview, and assessment that may influence how you go about discharge teaching for diabetes management?

7. How does your cultural assessment of Carmen Gonzales factor into your discharge teaching?

8. After considering the subjective and objective data for Carmen Gonzales, develop a list of nursing diagnoses and collaborative problems below. Include goals and possible interventions for each diagnosis or problem. Compare your problem list with information provided in the Ambulatory and Home Care section of your textbook. In what way does this plan of care relate to Carmen Gonzales' needs? What adaptations need to be made?

Nursing Diagnosis or Collaborative Problem	Goals	Interventions

→ Go to the discharge planning meeting today (see the bulletin board in the Nurses' Station for location). Also, read the health team reports in Carmen Gonzales' chart.

9. What types of needs does Carmen Gonzales have for dietary management related to her type 2 DM?

10. Below is a diagram representing the general dietary strategy for patients with type 2 diabetes. Using data you have gathered from Carmen Gonzales and information from your textbook, make specific suggestions to the patient related to each of the boxes in the diagram. Write your ideas directly on the diagram.

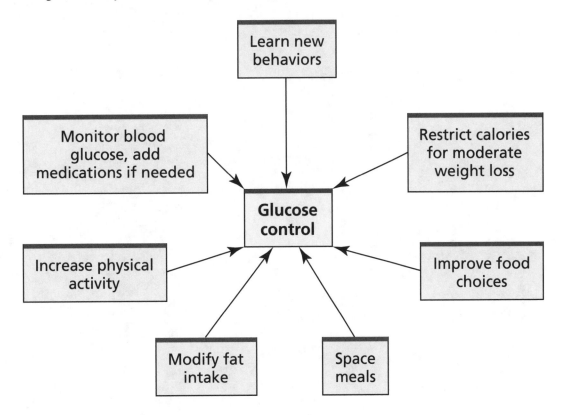

LESSON **26** ——————————————————————

Closed Head Injury

🕮 **Reading Assignment:** Nursing Assessment: Nervous System (Chapter 54)
Nursing Management: Intracranial Problems (Chapter 55)
Patient: David Ruskin, Room 303

For this lesson, you will study the case of David Ruskin, a 31-year-old male admitted to the hospital following a bicycle accident. He has been diagnosed with a closed head injury, fractured right humerus, and scalp laceration.

💿 **CD-ROM Activity**

Go to the Supervisor's Office and sign in to work with David Ruskin for the Tuesday 0700 shift. Proceed to the Nurses' Station and open his chart. Read the Emergency Department (ED) Report in the Physical & History section.

1. According to the Emergency Department Report, what was the mechanism of injury for David Ruskin? What other data are important to note regarding the accident and events immediately after the accident?

2. What was David Ruskin's neurologic status upon arrival to the ED?

3. What is the Glasgow Coma Scale? What are the three components of this scale? What does David Ruskin's score mean?

 Following a head injury, the physician's initial concern is cerebral edema and increased intracranial pressure (ICP). Answer the following questions related to these concepts. Refer to your textbook for help, if necessary.

4. What can cause cerebral edema following a head injury?

5. How does cerebral edema lead to ICP? What is the mechanism of increased ICP?

6. An immediate action by the Emergency Department staff was to administer high-flow oxygen to David Ruskin. Why was this done?

Review the content in the textbook regarding complications of head injury.

7. If David Ruskin has suffered a severe head injury resulting in increased ICP, what symptoms should you expect to see?

8. Two diagnostic tests were conducted in the Emergency Department to gain further information regarding David Ruskin's head injury: CT scan and skull series. What is the difference between these two tests? Why were these ordered?

Test	Description of Test and Reason Ordered
CT scan	
Skull series	

9. What were the results of the CT scan and skull series?

10. What is the main problem associated with CT scan for a patient who is not fully oriented? What can be done to help alleviate this problem?

→ Return to David Ruskin's chart and open the physicians' orders.

11. Read the postoperative orders for David Ruskin. Which orders specifically reflect the closed head injury diagnosis?

12. How are vital signs an important aspect of monitoring a patient with a closed head injury?

13. According to the physicians' orders, the nurses are to do "neuro checks." What should be included?

→ Now open the nurses' notes. Read the notes for Sunday and Monday.

14. What references are made in the documentation related to neurologic status?

→ Close the patient's chart and check the bulletin board to see where the night nurse is giving report on David Ruskin. Go to that location and listen to report.

15. What pertinent information related to David Ruskin's neurologic status is given in report?

16. What, if any, information did you find confusing during report? Is there anything else you would have liked the nurse to have included in the report? If so, what?

→ Now go into David Ruskin's room, click on **Vital Signs**, and obtain a set of vital sign readings.

17. Record David Ruskin's vital sign readings below. Then go to one of the computers that allow you to access the EPR and record them there as well.

Temperature _____   Respiration _____

Blood pressure _____   Oxygen saturation _____

Heart rate _____   Pain rating _____

→ Click on **Health History**, then on **Cognitive/Perceptual**, and listen to David Ruskin's responses in all three question areas. When you are finished, return to his chart in the Nurses' Station. Read through the Physical & History again, this time paying attention for data related to neurologic function.

18. Based on the data in these two areas, what can you document regarding the following neurologic findings?

Mental status

Pupil response/size

Glascow Coma Scale

Motor strength

Other cranial nerves assessed

LESSON 26—CLOSED HEAD INJURY

19. It has been 36 hours since David Ruskin's injury. Based on your assessment findings, indicate for each of the following possible types of head injury whether you think it is likely or unlikely that David Ruskin has this type of injury.

Epidural hematoma:

Acute subdural hematoma:

Subacute subdural hematoma:

20. Based on your answer to question 19, explain why this type of injury is still possible and how you might assess for it.

Acute Spinal Cord Injury— Part I: Preclinical Preparation

Reading Assignment: Nursing Management: Peripheral Nerve and Spinal Cord Problems (Chapter 59)

Patient: Andrea Wang, Room 310

For this lesson, you will complete preclinical preparation for Andrea Wang, a 20-year-old female who was admitted to the hospital a week ago following an acute spinal cord injury. The day of the injury, the patient went to emergency surgery and spent a week in ICU. On Monday of this week, she was transferred to the medical-surgical unit.

CD-ROM Activity

Go to the Supervisor's Office and sign in to work with Andrea Wang for the Tuesday 0700 shift. Proceed to the Nurses' Station and open her chart. Read the entire Physical & History, including the Emergency Department Record. (Remember to scroll down to read all pages.)

1. According to the Emergency Department Record, what was the mechanism of injury for Andrea Wang?

2. What are Andrea Wang's initial neurologic examination findings?

Area	Findings
Pupils	
Glasgow Coma Scale	
Orientation	
Cranial nerves	
Peripheral nerves	

3. Several radiographic diagnostic studies were performed in the Emergency Department, including a chest x-ray and an MRI. According to the Emergency Department Record, what do these studies reveal?

Read about spinal cord trauma in your textbook.

4. Describe the pathophysiology of spinal cord trauma during the acute or initial injury stage.

5. Why is spinal edema such a serious concern following an acute spinal cord injury?

6. Which of the following pictures represents the type of spinal injury Andrea Wang has suffered? Circle the correct answer.

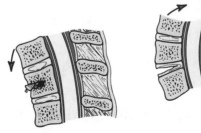

Flexion injury   **Extension injury**

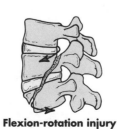   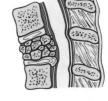

Flexion-rotation injury   **Compression injury**

7. According to the Emergency Department Record, Andrea Wang has a partially transected spinal cord at T6. What does *partial transection* mean?

8. What are the six types of syndromes associated with incomplete lesions of the spinal cord?

   a.

   b.

   c.

   d.

   e.

   f.

9. Which of the six syndromes from question 8 do you suspect Andrea Wang is experiencing? Why?

10. The physician indicates that Andrea Wang also suffers from spinal shock. Describe spinal shock.

11. According to the Emergency Department Record, a Foley catheter was inserted in the Emergency Department. What, if anything, does this have to do with Andrea Wang's spinal cord injury?

12. The physician's plan also included "steroid protocol for spinal injury." What drug is typically used for this? What is the usual dose, and how is it given in this situation? What benefit does this provide? (You may need to refer to a drug handbook.)

Drug	Typical Dose and Administration	Beneficial Effects

13. Andrea Wang was sent to the OR for decompression and fusion of the thoracic spine within 1 1/2 hours of arrival. What is the purpose of this surgical procedure, and why was it done immediately?

→ In Andrea Wang's chart, click on **Physicians' Orders** and review the orders for Monday (*not including medication orders*).

14. Indicate the rationale for the physician's orders. (If you need help, consult the Care Plan in your textbook.)

Orders (not including medications)	Rationale

Close Andrea Wang's chart and open the MAR (in the blue notebook on the counter).

15. Examine the list of medications Andrea Wang is receiving. Why are they being given?

Medication	Classification	Reason Given
Famotidine 20 mg PO q12h		
Docusate sodium 100 mg PO qd		
Biscodyl suppository 10 mg, QOD PRN		
Multiple vitamin with minerals qAM		
Vitamin C 500 mg PO qPM		
Enoxaparin 30 mg SC q12h		
Baclofen 10 mg PO q12h		
Acetaminophen 600 mg PO q4–6h PRN		
Oxycodone/ acetominophen 1 tablet PO PRN		

→ Close the MAR and return to Andrea Wang's chart. Click on **Nurses' Notes**. As you read the notes, consider the major concerns that emerge regarding this patient's care.

16. Create a list of concerns and a problem list based on the data you have collected thus far from the chart.

 a. Concerns:

 b. Problem list (nursing diagnoses and collaborative problems):

LESSON 28

Acute Spinal Cord Injury— Part II

📖 **Reading Assignment:** Nursing Management: Peripheral Nerve and Spinal Cord
Problems (Chapter 59)

Patient: Andrea Wang, Room 310

For this lesson, you will continue to care for Andrea Wang, a 20-year-old female admitted to the hospital following an acute spinal cord injury. You should have completed Lesson 27 prior to beginning this lesson.

💿 **CD-ROM Activity**

Go to the Supervisor's Office and sign in to work with Andrea Wang for the Tuesday 0700 shift. Proceed to the bulletin board in the Nurses' Station and find the location of the nursing report. (Remember: you can also find this information by moving your cursor across the animated map in the upper right corner of your screen.)

1. Listen to report and record pertinent notes below.

2. Did anything in the report seem inconsistent? Is there anything else you wish the nurse would have addressed during report? Explain.

→ Go to Andrea Wang's room and click on **Vital Signs**.

3. Take a set of vital sign readings, including pain rating. Record these below and in the EPR.

Heart rate _____   Temperature _____

Respiratory rate _____   Oxygen saturation _____

Blood pressure _____   Pain rating/location _____

4. Based on Andrea Wang's vital signs, what nursing intervention is appropriate?

→ Next, click on **Physical**.

5. Collect all the physical examination data for Andrea Wang and record below and on the next page. Are any data out of the ordinary and/or unexpected?

Area Examined	Findings
Head and Neck	
Chest/Upper Extremities	

Area Examined	Findings
Abdomen and Lower Extremities	

→ Click on **Medications** and then on **Administer**. Observe the nurse give Andrea Wang her 0900 medications.

    6. Which routine medication due at 0900 did the nurse fail to administer?

→ Click on **Health History** and conduct a complete interview.

    7. As you listen to the interview for each of the 12 health history categories, record significant data below and on the next page.

Area	Significant Data
Perception/Self-Concept	
Activity	

Area	Significant Data
Sexuality/Reproduction	
Culture	
Nutrition-Metabolic	
Sleep-Rest	
Role/Relationship	

Area	Significant Data
Health Perception	
Elimination	
Cognitive/Perceptual	
Coping/Stress	
Value/Belief	

8. Now that you have collected data from the health history, the physical examination, and vital sign readings, revisit the problem list you developed in Lesson 27 (question 16b). Record that list in the left column below. Based on what you have learned, revise your list in the right column.

Original Problem List (from Lesson 27)	New Revised Problem List
Nursing diagnoses:	Nursing diagnoses:
Collaborative problems:	Collaborative problems:

→ We will now make a virtual leap in time to Thursday. To do this, return to the Supervisor's Office and sign in again on the desktop computer. Click on **Reset** and select Andrea Wang for Thursday 1100. Next, find the location of the nursing report on Andrea Wang. Go to that location and listen to report.

9. Record significant data from report below.

→ Now click on **Health Team Meeting** and listen to these reports on Andrea Wang.

10. Below, record the primary concerns of each of the health team members. When you have
finished, go to the Nurses' Station and open Andrea Wang's chart. Click on **Health Team**,
read each member's report, and add additional data below.

Case Manager

Social Worker

Clinical Nurse
Specialist

11. The clinical nurse specialist and other nurses mention the need to monitor Andrea Wang for autonomic dysreflexia. What is this? What are the symptoms? How is this condition managed?

→ Click on **Nurses' Notes** and read the notes since Tuesday.

12. From the nurses' notes, what issues are evident regarding Andrea Wang's care?

13. You are asked to spend time with Andrea Wang going over measures to prevent skin break-down. Write down some ideas you have regarding what you should discuss with her. Refer to your textbook for ideas.

→ We will once again make a virtual leap in time and jump ahead to Friday. Return to the Supervisor's Office and sign in to work with Andrea Wang for the Friday shift. Proceed to the Nurses' Station and open her chart.

14. Read the nurses' notes from Thursday night. What complication developed?

15. What was the apparent cause of the complication?

16. Were Andrea Wang's symptoms consistent with those presented in the textbook? What were her symptoms?

Skeletal Fracture

 Reading Assignment: Nursing Assessment: Musculoskeletal System (Chapter 60)
Nursing Management: Musculoskeletal Trauma and Orthopedic Surgery (Chapter 61)

Patient: David Ruskin, Room 303

For this lesson, you are assigned to care for David Ruskin, a 31-year-old male patient who was hit by a car while riding his bike. This patient has, among many injuries, a fracture to his right arm.

CD-ROM Activity

Go to the Supervisor's Office and sign in to work with David Ruskin for Tuesday at 0700. Proceed to the Nurses' Station and open the patient's chart. Read the entire Physical & History, including the Emergency Department Report. (Remember to scroll down to read all pages.)

1. According to your textbook, the initial clinical manifestations of a fractured humerus can include the following: edema, bone deformity, decreased bone function, pain, ecchymosis, and crepitation. Describe the significance of those clinical findings below and on the next page. Then, compare these typical clinical findings with those described for David Ruskin in the Emergency Department Report. Circle those findings that are documented.

Clinical Finding	Significance
Edema	
Decreased function	

Clinical Finding	Significance
Pain	
Ecchymosis	
Crepitation	

2. What additional data were included in the Emergency Department Report regarding the fractured humerus?

3. If you had done the initial ED assessment of the right arm, what additional data might you have included?

Now consider all the presenting injuries as documented in the Emergency Department Report. Consider how you would have prioritized your assessment if you had been working in the ER when David Ruskin was brought in.

4. Below, list all of David Ruskin's presenting injuries in the first column. In the second column, rank each injury according to what you believe to be the priority of assessment (highest = 1; next highest = 2, etc.) In the third column, indicate what impact these other injuries may have had on assessment of the fractured humerus (if any).

Presenting Injury	Priority of Assessment	Impact of Injury on Assessment of the Arm (if any)

Click on **Diagnostics** in David Ruskin's chart. Read the x-ray report for Sunday at 1600.

5. Based on Dr. Kawasaki's report, circle the picture below that best represents the type of fracture David Ruskin has?

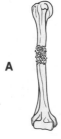
A

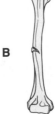
B

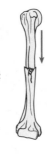
C

→ Now click on **Physicians' Orders** and review the orders for Sunday night through Tuesday morning. When you are finished, close the chart and access the patient's MAR (in the blue notebook on the counter.) Review David Ruskin's MAR.

6. Determine what routine medication(s) you will be giving to David Ruskin today during the day shift (0700–1500). Below, list the medication(s) you need to give, the reason why each is given, and the time each is due.

Medication	Why Given	Time Due

→ The night nurse is ready to start report on David Ruskin. Close the MAR, check the bulletin for location, and go to hear report.

7. Record significant data from report below.

8. What did you think about the report you were given? Were there any inconsistencies? Is there anything else you wish the nurse would have included in the report related to the fractured arm?

 9. Formulate a care plan for the day. Refer to Nursing Care Plan 61-1 in your textbook and review the nursing care plan for a patient with a fracture. Below, list what you consider to be the top five priority nursing diagnoses and/or collaborative problem(s) from Nursing Care Plan 61-1 that are applicable in this clinical situation (with the focus on the fractured humerus). In the second column, list some of the interventions you think would be appropriate for David Ruskin.

**Nursing Diagnosis
or
Collaborative Problem**   **Intervention**

→ Go to David Ruskin's room and obtain a set of vital signs.

10. Record David Ruskin's vital signs below and then enter them in the EPR.

Heart rate _____   Temperature _____

Respiratory rate _____   Oxygen saturation _____

Blood pressure _____

→ In David Ruskin's room, click on **Physical** and conduct a complete bedside examination.

11. Below, record your findings from David Ruskin's physical examination.

Area Examined	Findings
Head and Neck	
Chest/Upper Extremities	
Abdomen and Lower Extremities	

12. Consider all the data you have just collected. What interventions might you provide at this time? Is there anything missing? Is there anything that changes your plan of care?

→ A nursing assistant tells you that David Ruskin seems to be in pain. Go to his room and assess the situation. First, obtain his pain rating. Then go to one of the computers that access the EPR and record his pain level there.

13. What medication(s) can be given to David Ruskin for the pain? What other data need to be assessed before you make a decision to give him a pain medication at this time?

Pain rating = _____

Medication(s) available:

Other symptoms:

Decision (choose one):

___ Medicate David Ruskin with _____

___ Do not medicate David Ruskin at this time.

Rationale:

→ It is time to give David Ruskin his 0900 medications. Go to his room and administer the medications.

Lunch time! Leave the floor and go to lunch.

→ After lunch, sign in again to work with David Ruskin for Tuesday 1100. Go to the Nurses' Station and access the patient's MAR. Note that David Ruskin has cefoxitin due at 1200. Before you give the medication, consider a few things about this drug. (You will probably want to refer to a drug handbook.)

14. What is the purpose of cefoxitin?

15. In what types of IV solution could you expect the cefoxitin to be diluted? (In other words, with what IV solutions is it compatible?)

16. How long should it take to administer 1 gram of cefoxitin?

→ Now access David Ruskin's EPR and find his CBC results.

17. What is David Ruskin's WBC count result?

18. What does this result mean?

→ Check David Ruskin's body temperature trends over the last several days.

19. What do you see happening with his body temperature?

20. How are David Ruskin's WBC count and his temperature trends relevant in regard to giving him cefoxitin?

LESSON 30 —————————————————————————

Osteomyelitis

———————————————————————————————

Reading Assignment: Nursing Management: Musculoskeletal Problems (Chapter 62)
Patient: Carmen Gonzales, Room 302

For this lesson, you are assigned to care for Carmen Gonzales, a 56-year-old female patient admitted to the hospital with type 2 diabetes mellitus, a leg infection, and osteomyelitis.

 Before you begin, review the etiology and pathophysiology of osteomyelitis in your textbook.

  1. What does the term *osteomyelitis* mean?

  2. What is the difference between acute and chronic osteomyelitis?

   Acute osteomyelitis

   Chronic osteomyelitis

3. Osteomyelitis can occur by direct or indirect invasion. Describe the difference.

Direct invasion

Indirect invasion

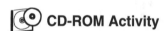 **CD-ROM Activity**

Go to the Supervisor's Office and sign in to work with Carmen Gonzales for the Tuesday 0700 shift. Proceed to the Nurses' Station and open her chart. Read the entire Physical & History, including the Emergency Department Record. (Scroll down to read all pages.)

4. The clinical manifestations of osteomyelitis can include both local and systemic symptoms. Common local and systemic signs and symptoms are listed below. Circle signs and symptoms consistent with Carmen Gonzales' history and physical examination findings on admission.

Local Symptoms	Systemic Symptoms
Severe bone pain	Fever
Swelling	Night sweats
Warmth at infection site	Chills
Restricted movement	Restlessness
	Nausea
	Malaise

5. Based on what you have read, identify the source of Carmen Gonzales' osteomyelitis and the type of invasion responsible for it.

Type of Invasion (circle one)	**Source**
Direct Indirect	

→ Now click on **Physicians' Orders** and read the orders for Sunday evening.

6. The following diagnostic tests are useful in the diagnosis and evaluation of osteomyelitis. Match each test with its corresponding description. Then circle Yes or No to indicate whether or not each diagnostic test was performed as part of Carmen Gonzales' admissions work-up.

	Diagnostic Test	**Description**
Yes No _____	MRI and CT scan	a. Initial test to determine causative organism.
Yes No _____	Wound culture	
Yes No _____	Blood leukocyte count	b. Helpful to identify boundaries of the infection.
Yes No _____	X-ray of affected extremity	c. Most definitive way to determine causative organism.
Yes No _____	Radionuclide bone scan	
Yes No _____	Bone/tissue biopsy	d. Elevated results of this test indicate infection.

e. Radiologic test that can identify osteomyelitis within 72 hours of onset.

f. Changes with this test do not appear until at least 10 days after onset of clinical symptoms.

➡ Click on **Diagnostics** and review the radiologic report for Sunday at 1600 hours. Compare this report with the pathophysiology of osteomyelitis as described in the textbook.

7. What finding is documented on the x-ray report that is consistent with osteomyelitis? What does this finding mean?

Finding documented on the x-ray report

Meaning

➡ Click on **Surgeons' Notes** and review the surgical report for Monday afternoon.

8. According to the textbook, collaborative care of osteomyelitis may include surgical debridement of the bony tissue. What type of surgery was performed in Carmen Gonzales' case? Did this include surgical debridement of the bone?

→ Now close the chart and go to the MAR in the blue notebook on the counter. Open Carmen Gonzales' MAR for today.

9. Determine what routine medication(s) (including the continuous IV) you will be giving to Carmen Gonzales today during the day shift (0700–1500). Below, list the medication(s) you need to give, the reason why each is given, and the time each is due.

Medication	Why Given	Time Due

→ You are aware that the cefoxitin has been ordered for Carmen Gonzales because of her leg infection. You decide to check the WBC done on Sunday night because you are curious (also, you are sure your nursing instructor will ask you about it). Close the MAR and go to the computer under the bookshelf to access the EPR. Find the hematology results for Carmen Gonzales.

10. Below, record Carmen Gonzales' hematology results for Sunday night. Explain what each result means.

Test	Result	What does this mean?
Hgb		
Hct		
WBC		

➡ The night nurse is ready to give report on Carmen Gonzales. Close the EPR, check the bulletin board for report location, and go to hear the report.

11. Record significant data from the report below.

12. What did you think about the report you were given? Is there anything else you wish the nurse would have included in the report regarding osteomyelitis? If so, what?

➡ It is now 0745. Go to Carmen Gonzales' room, click on **Vital Signs**, and obtain a full set of vital sign readings.

13. Record Carmen Gonzales' vital sign readings below and in the EPR.

Heart rate _____   Temperature _____

Respiratory rate _____   Oxygen saturation _____

Blood pressure _____   Pain rating _____

14. Based on what you have learned from obtaining Carmen Gonzales' vital signs, you should return to her room to give her what PRN medication? Why?

→ Carmen Gonzales is due to receive cefoxitin at 0800. The pharmacy sends premixed cefoxitin IV. The label reads "2 grams cefoxitin in 50 ml D_5W." Answer the following questions regarding the administration of IV cefoxitin. (You may want to refer to a nursing drug handbook.)

15. Is this IV cefoxitin solution compatible with the primary IV infusion?

16. Over what amount of time should you infuse this IV antibiotic?

17. If you are using an IV pump to deliver this medication piggyback, what rate (mL per hour) will you select to give this infusion?

    _____ mL/hour

→ Now return to Carmen Gonzales' room and conduct a complete physical examination and health history.

18. After gathering data from the health history interview and physical examination, develop a plan of care for the day for Carmen Gonzales. Refer to Nursing Care Plan 62-1 in your textbook. Complete each of the nursing diagnoses on the next two pages by tailoring them to Carmen Gonzales' situation. Provide goals and interventions for each diagnosis.

Nursing Diagnosis

Acute pain related to

_____

as manifested by

_____

Impaired physical mobility related to

_____

as manifested by

_____

Goal(s)

Interventions

Nursing Diagnosis	Goal(s)	Interventions
Ineffective therapeutic regimen management related to _____ as manifested by _____		

➡️ Go to the Supervisor's Office and sign in again to work with Carmen Gonzales—this time for the Thursday 1100 shift.

📖 You are interested in Carmen Gonzales' discharge needs related to the osteomyelitis. Attend the health team meeting and listen to each member's report. Then go to the Nurses' Station and read the health team reports in Carmen Gonzales' chart. Finally, refer to the Ambulatory and Home Care section of your textbook.

19. Based on what you know and have read, what do you expect will be included in Carmen Gonzales' discharge instructions and follow-up care to manage her osteomyelitis?

Notes